YOGA

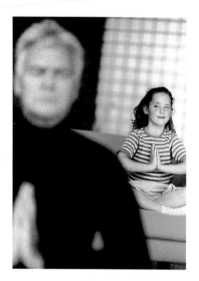

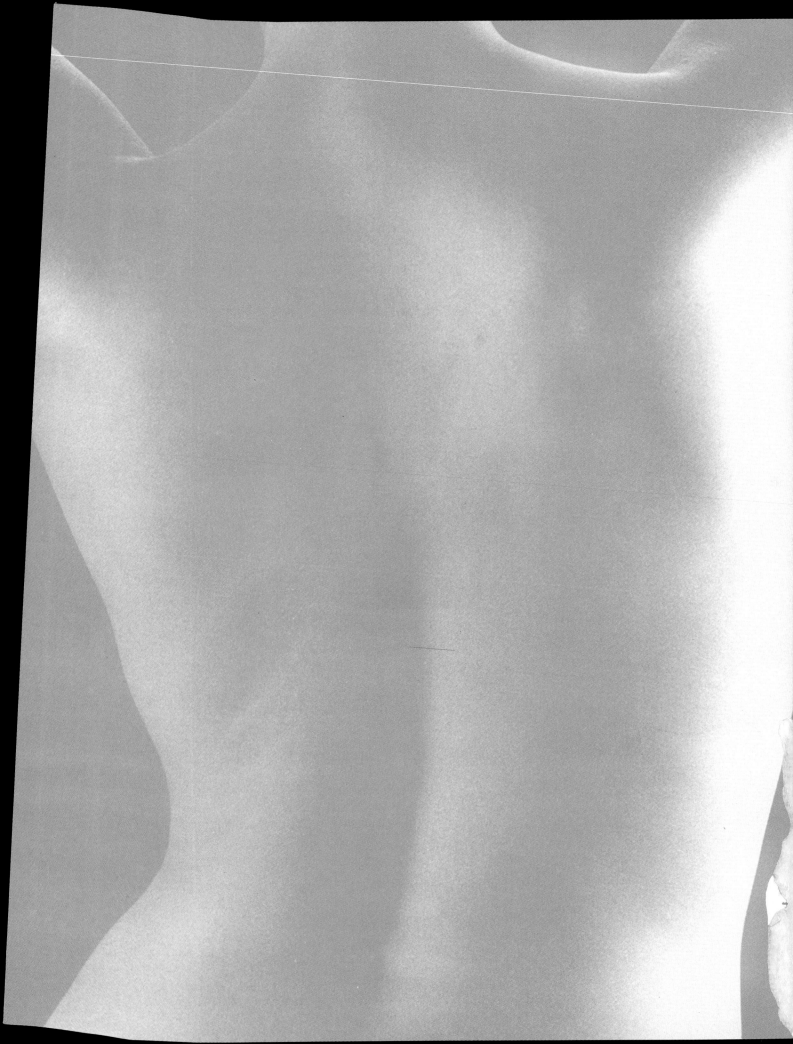

an introduction to
YOGA

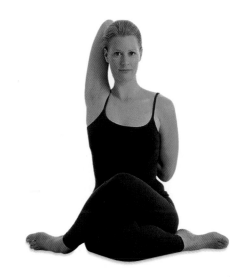

Christina Brown

This is a Parragon book
This edition published in 2005

Parragon
Queen Street House
4 Queen Street
Bath BA1 1HE, UK

Copyright © Parragon 2002

This book was created by
THE BRIDGEWATER BOOK COMPANY

Photography Senthil Kumar

A CIP catalogue record for this book is
available from the British Library

ISBN 1-40544-622-6

Printed in Indonesia

Contents

Introduction

Yoga is not merely a series of exercises simultaneously energising and relaxing the body, it is a means of harmonising the mind, body and spirit and is a great tool of transformation.

Om asathoma satgamaya

Thamasoma Jyotirgamaya

Mrithyorma Amrithangamaya

Om Shanti Shanti Shanti

Om Lead me from the unreal to the real

From darkness to light

From the predicament of death, to immortality

Om peace, peace, peace

Sanskrit chant

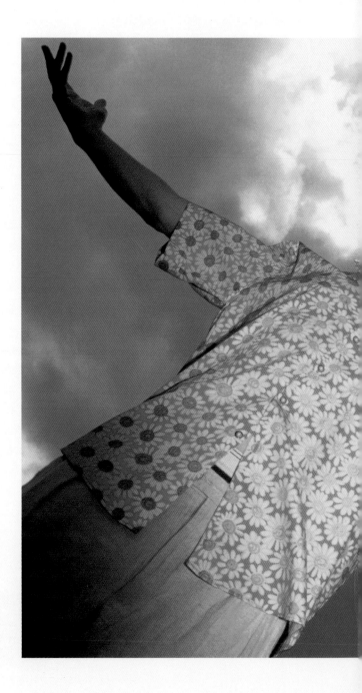

In the *chitta-vrtti*, a text that codifies the subject, yoga is defined as *chitta-vrtti-nirohdah*, the cessation of the fluctuations of the mind. Yoga is actually a state of being, not an exercise or a physical posture.

The aim of yoga is to separate the spirit within from the physical body which acts as its vessel. As the yoga practitioner seeks control over the mind, the thoughts are stilled and the yogi's essential purity is regained. This neutralisation of the turnings of thought occurs in a trance-like state known as *samadhi*.

Asana, the use of physical postures, is the practice most commonly equated with yoga in the west. Asana helps to open and prepare the body for the long hours of meditation necessary to reach this goal. It also alters the subtle energies of the body, clearing the path for the experience of higher states.

An energy known as the *kundalini* resides in the body. Literally translated as 'she who is coiled', the kundalini force is likened to a serpent said to lie dormant at the base of the spine. It is this reservoir of energy that Hatha yoga practice, including asanas, seeks to awaken. Hatha yoga purifies the body and mind to clear the way for this cosmic power. Yoga asanas stretch and irrigate the spine to encourage the upward movement of the kundalini.

The word *yoga* originates from the Sanskrit *yug*, meaning 'to yoke'. Yoking, or harnessing energies, implies effort, and a goal such as *samadhi* certainly requires discipline. Though the starting point for many people is a few yoga postures, Hatha yoga, sometimes referred to as the 'yoga of force', also includes codes of moral conduct, asanas, breathing practices, concentration and meditation. These are the tools to achieve union with the cosmic universal power and the state of yoga.

Self-realisation and entering samadhi are lofty goals indeed. More realistically, yoga practice has a lot to offer us in the 21st century. *Yug* is also translated as 'to link or unify'. Even while attempting to disunite – to isolate spirit from matter – yoga practice gives a subjective feeling of union. It helps to harmonize the mind, body and spirit. By connecting thought, breath and posture, yoga aligns the mental, physical and emotional bodies. Yoga practice offers a chance to return to the integrated self and experience the truth of who we are. In experiencing these mini self-realisations we get a glimpse of our essential purity. It is like remembering who we really are, but, caught up in the whirlwind of life, had forgotten.

Every yoga practice is a small reversal of consciousness. Yoga teaches us to quieten the mind and observe the present moment. In a refreshing way, our minds are jolted out of our everyday way of thinking. It teaches patience and humbleness in the face of difficulty. We learn to respond to challenges. Yoga expands the heart and gives a sense of wholeness and peace. It is a tremendous tool for transformation.

LEFT *Yoga will help you to achieve a feeling of unity.*

BELOW *Practising yoga teaches an ability to quieten the mind.*

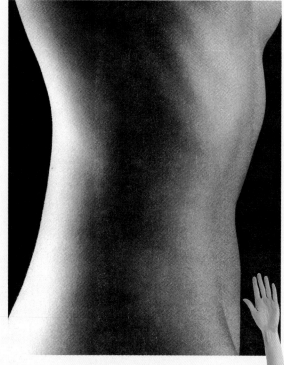

Attention to correct alignment during yoga practice can improve overall body posture.

ASANA AND ALIGNMENT

Yoga postures are based on ancient geometrical shapes. When performed with attention to alignment, these asanas redesign the body. Muscles are trained to lengthen out of their habitual tense, shortened holding patterns. Sometimes a tight area of the body is compensating for another weaker area. This area of higher tension can finally lessen this protective holding as the weaker zone strengthens. Even bones can and do change shape over time. Bone cells are constantly broken down and new cells laid down where they will best sustain the force of the most common daily impacts. Often we are not fully aware of how we hold and carry ourselves. To help undo less than optimal holding patterns, attend classes with an experienced teacher who can give feedback on your alignment.

Asanas assist the rhythmic pulsations of the body. Blood and cerebrospinal fluid circulation, digestion, excretion, lymphatic drainage and all the organs require rhythmic pulsation to maintain good health. Yoga postures, by freeing up the body for these natural pulsations, aid good health. Practising yoga postures is like giving yourself a massage, not just to the muscles, but to the deeper tissues and internal organs too. Asanas are a great form of do-it-yourself preventative medicine.

Asanas work on more than just a physical level. They take the intelligence normally considered to reside in the mind and spread it throughout the entire body. Consciousness can reach everywhere. In the perfect asana, the mind is so engrossed that there is no room for other thoughts to arise. Asanas have psycho-spiritual effects. They influence the emotions and express qualities of the heart.

By aligning the outer body, asanas improve the energy flow in the inner body. Asanas help keep, build and control the vital force, the *prana*.

Spread mental focus from one part of the body to another to develop a simultaneous overall awareness.

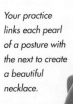

Your practice links each pearl of a posture with the next to create a beautiful necklace.

One of the most common mental blocks for a beginner is the belief that they are not flexible enough for yoga. However, if you perform a pose with honest effort and correct alignment, you will achieve a result similar to that of someone who seems more flexible. Do not despair about your lack of flexibility; the true measure of your asana is being mentally present – aware of the whole body – and having a calm and steady breath.

BREATHING

The mind and breath are interrelated; an alteration in one affects the other. By nature, the breath is more constant than the mind. The mind can multiply in ways the breath cannot. Focusing on the breath in asana practice helps to calm the consciousness. For this reason, never force the breath. Inhalations and exhalations are like waves breaking on the shore. Keep them even to develop evenness in the mind.

Conscious breathing in a pose will deepen your awareness and keep your mind free of distraction. The breath is your monitor of how you are doing in the pose. When the breath is perfectly steady, your asana is closer to being perfected.

Breathe through the nose not the mouth, so the air is filtered and warmed. Perform asanas with Ujjayi breathing (see page 83). As a general rule, inhale when you come up out of a pose, when raising the arms, and during movements that expand the chest such as bending backwards. Exhale when moving downwards, lowering the arms or bending forwards.

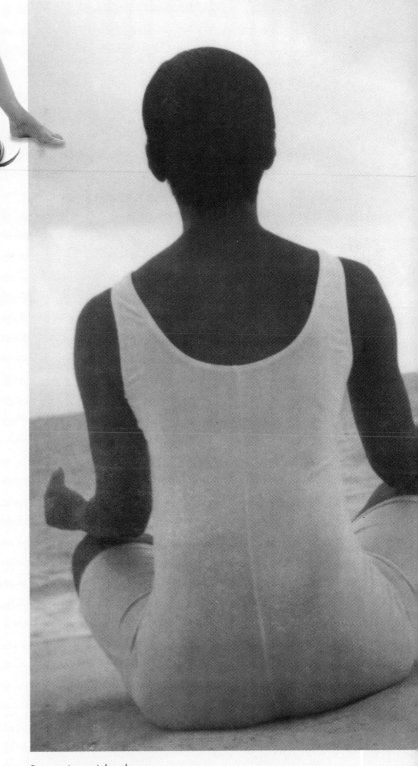

For centuries, yogis have known that calming the breath helps to quieten the mind.

AWARENESS, FOCUS AND BEING PRESENT

When an asana is performed with full awareness, it develops into something far greater than just a fitness regime. Work with integrity. Become absorbed in the subtle sensations of the body. From observing your hamstring in a forward bend, for example, spread your awareness to the whole leg, then to your lower back without forgetting the original point, radiate your awareness out until it touches the entire body. The essence of yoga is not about twisting yourself into complicated pretzel shapes. Doing the most difficult looking asanas is not the goal. Rather, mastery of an asana comes when a perfect awareness of the whole body and breath can be maintained.

Working consciously focuses your attention right at the present moment. You may spend one minute in a posture. During this minute, you let go, observe and refine, seeking the still point, the epicentre of consciousness. During yoga, these minutes link together. If each asana is a pearl, an asana practice forms a beautiful necklace.

Over time, this 'one minute' focus can extend into your day-to-day life. Yoga is practising being in the 'now'. Give attention to the breath, which will bring you back to the present. When you are fully in the present, worries about the future dissipate. Stress floats away when you can release the past and let go of concerns for the future.

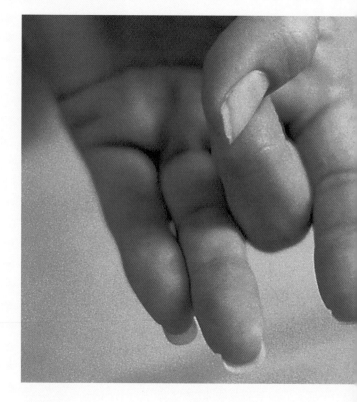

EFFORT

Fully engaging a muscle helps to bring the mind right to that area. Engaging a muscle group increases awareness and is good practice for concentration and being in the now. When the muscles are engaged, the mind is engaged – one reason why asanas have transformative power. The effort required teaches discipline and is rewarding.

For beginners, holding a posture might require 90% effort. It is hard to feel the surrender and release that is the other 10%. With time and dedication, this percentage shifts. The asana becomes more comfortable and feels more rewarding, as the effort it demands falls to 80%, then 70% and so on. Experiencing the freedom in the pose by yielding into it is sweetly satisfying.

There needs to be a balance between effort and surrender. If you don't extend yourself fully, the practice will be too easy, and your attention will

Yoga is practising being in the 'now'. Focus on your breathing to bring your attention to the present.

from your lungs, release the tension in the body. Don't force it. To extend further, yield with each exhalation. Use rhythm to help you relax into the poses. If you have difficulty getting a sensation of release in a pose, use external movement. Move in and out of the pose with a rhythmic flow several times before holding the pose steady.

FINDING THE EDGE

Learning to extend yourself to the limit requires experimentation to find just where the frontier lies. It changes daily, so you have to rediscover the edge in each pose of every practice. Metaphysically, reaching your edge and nudging your boundaries challenges your perception of where you are at. Yoga asanas are a controlled means of exposing yourself to a difficult situation. They are meant to try you. They offer practice at not being stressed in stressful conditions.

A single posture will have many edges. As you arrive at the first one, stay steady and breathe for a while. Have patience. Wait for the posture to let you in. When it does, enter respectfully. Again hold and breathe at this new edge, waiting for the invitation from your body to enter.

As you approach your 'edge', distinguish between discomfort and pain. On the road to strength, flexibility and focus, mental and physical unease inevitably arises. Discomfort is just resistance of the body or mind. Don't fight physical unease, but soften into it. For mental unease, become absorbed by the breath to return to the present.

Pain is more acute than discomfort. Pain in a pose means you have approached your edge too fast and gone too far or that you are improperly aligned. Pain in the muscles or joints should not be ignored because it can lead to injury. Come out of the pose and examine your alignment. Consult a teacher if necessary. In time you will become more body aware and better able to listen to feedback from your body.

wander. When you overextend yourself, it becomes so difficult that your practice will not be joyful. Practising with effort doesn't mean using excess force. Frowning, clenching your jaw or holding your breath are signs to back off. If you feel competitive, smile kindly upon yourself, and let go of your over-ambitiousness. Your practice is a metaphor for life. Delight in it.

SURRENDER

Life experiences build up like layers and are stored in the cellular memory of our bodies. The asanas allow you to explore and soften the unconscious holding on. Yoga helps us to strip off the superfluous emotional overlays that hold us back. There is a sense of freedom and peace within at discovering our true essence.

We are accustomed to the concept of using effort to get somewhere. Letting go in order to achieve something might seem strange. Yoga uses effort – doing – to aid surrender – undoing. With yoga you can often do more by undoing. As you release the air

GROUNDING

If you want one part of your body to rise up, you must anchor another part down. Each pose has an anchor point. Working from this base teaches you how to extend yourself, while not losing yourself. When no attention is given to grounding, yoga poses risk turning into a series of mere stretches.

Often less flexible people practise better yoga than very flexible ones, because stiffer bodied people have more intuitive experience about anchoring and working from their base. Very 'stretchy' people sometimes find it hard to learn to anchor themselves. A certain amount of stability is always needed, both in life and in the poses. The earth supports, shelters and feeds us, yet sometimes we lose our sense of connection with it.

Re-centre, find your balance and extend yourself to your limit without losing awareness of what is always there to support you.

RESTING

Nobody would expect a car driven continuously, at high speed, not to deteriorate. Yet many of us expect it from our bodies. Relaxation during asana practice allows the body space to give the mind feedback. Awareness and intuition will develop. Until the art of relaxation *within* the postures is developed, rest when necessary between postures. See Relaxation Breaks (pages 74–85) for resting poses.

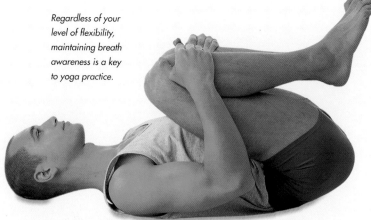

Regardless of your level of flexibility, maintaining breath awareness is a key to yoga practice.

HISTORY AND PHILOSOPHY

Many scholars date Hatha Yoga back to between the ninth and tenth centuries. However, the ideas and practices were passed down orally before being written down, so it is possible they are much older than this.

Yoga consists of eight limbs (see chart opposite), as codified in the *Yoga-sutras*. Written in Sanskrit and attributed to Patanjali, the *Yoga-sutras* is an early yoga text. Patanjali lists the eight limbs in a certain order, starting with moral behaviour and ending with the self-realised state of *samadhi*.

They are not steps to be worked on one by one, but branches to be explored several at a time – otherwise we would forever remain at the very first precept of the first limb – practicing only non-violence. Our whole lives would have to be lived without causing injury and we'd never move on to practising a single asana.

From a relatively simple beginning using asanas, yoga sometimes takes you by the hand and leads you on to the higher concepts. You have the support of a force greater than yourself, so it feels like a natural progression to explore some of the other limbs.

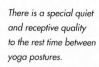

There is a special quiet and receptive quality to the rest time between yoga postures.

The first five limbs are known as the outer limbs. Limbs three, four and five involve the interpenetration of the mind, body and spirit. The last three limbs, the inner limbs, are called the 'wealth of yoga' by Patanjali. It's debatable whether you can 'practise' them or not because they are states of the mind. However, you can make yourself as receptive as possible to them.

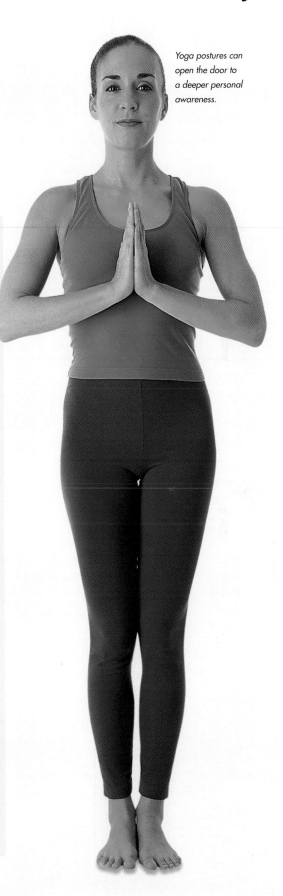

Yoga postures can open the door to a deeper personal awareness.

THE EIGHT LIMBS OF YOGA

1 YAMA Moral restraints. Five are listed in the *Yoga-sutras*: non-injury, truthfulness, non-stealing, chastity and non-covetousness.

2 NIYAMA Discipline in actions and conduct. Patanjali lists five disciplines: cleanliness, contentment, austerity, continuous learning and surrender to the Divine.

3 ASANA The physical postures of Hatha Yoga.

4 PRANAYAMA Breath control to cultivate the vital force within. For more information, see pages 16–17 and 80–85.

5 PRATYAHARA Withdrawal of the senses. An example of pratyahara might be when you are so engrossed in watching a movie that you don't hear a fire engine siren outside. The noise is still there but it is not consciously registered; the mind receives fewer distractions. Often, instead of us controlling the senses, the sense organs become masters over us. Like servants we drive five miles to satisfy the craving for a particular food. On the spiritual path, the mind gradually loses interest in what the senses have to say and pratyahara becomes more natural.

6 DHARANA Mental concentration. This can be practised during asana and pranayama practice. *Dharana* helps pave the way to the seventh and eighth limbs. It is the third step in the practice in the section on Meditation.

7 DHYANA As meditation, *dhyana* is a one-pointed mental focus (see pages 88–89).

8 SAMADHI Consciousness is altered in this illuminated state of absorption with the absolute.

Starting the practice

These guidelines will help you get the most from your practice session. Remember that in yoga it is important to focus on the journey, rather than just the destination.

Yoga makes energy available to the cells to repair and detoxify. Avoid diverting this energy into digestion. Don't practise on a full stomach. Wait four hours after a large meal before practising and leave half an hour after your practice before eating. Unless absolutely necessary, it's best to avoid drinking water during the practice.

When you are short of time, practising fewer poses with full attention is preferable to rushing through many poses. Each balanced practice will include a forward bend, side bend, back bend, twist, balance, inversion and a final relaxation. Always include a pose that makes you feel good about your practice, but include one you don't like so much, as that one is probably exactly what you need most.

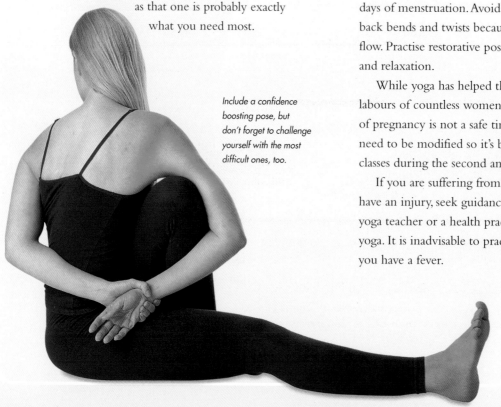

Include a confidence boosting pose, but don't forget to challenge yourself with the most difficult ones, too.

Practising twice a week is a good start. Three times a week heralds a deeper level of transformation. If your practice is intense, rest one day a week. If you miss a practice, your yoga space will never feel jilted or be upset with you when you return. It will always welcome you back.

Though the idea is lovely, practising in direct sunlight tends to be fatiguing. Choose a warm spot, with a clean, level surface. A cushioned surface is nice for some of the floor poses. Sticky mats offer cushioning and will prevent slipping in the standing postures. Choose clothes that let you stretch and that you feel good in.

Women should take things easy during the initial days of menstruation. Avoid inverted postures, strong back bends and twists because they can affect the flow. Practise restorative poses, such as forward bends and relaxation.

While yoga has helped the pregnancies and labours of countless women, the first three months of pregnancy is not a safe time to begin. Many poses need to be modified so it's best to attend specialised classes during the second and third trimesters.

If you are suffering from a health condition or have an injury, seek guidance from an experienced yoga teacher or a health practitioner who understands yoga. It is inadvisable to practise asana or pranayama if you have a fever.

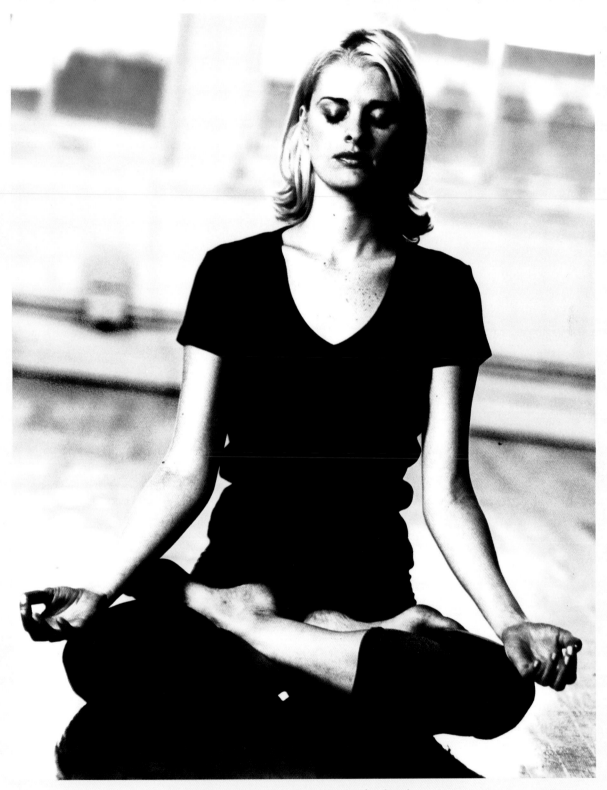

*Never rush your yoga practice. More benefit is derived
from taking more time over fewer postures than skipping
through a routine with less awareness.*

Awareness of the **breath**

When you practise yoga you are dedicating some time only to you. Unplug the telephone and close the door on distractions. You might light a candle. Honour yourself and the light you carry within. With regard to the outside energies greater than yourself, you could offer a prayer or chant. Begin lying down or sitting in order to access the stillness within. Quieten the mind and observe the present moment by focusing on your breath.

YOGIC THOUGHT
Yoga is both the journey and the endpoint.

1 Lie on your right side with your knees bent. Reach your arms straight out in front, palms together. Gaze at your left thumb and, inhaling, take your left arm up in the air until your fingers point straight up to the sky.

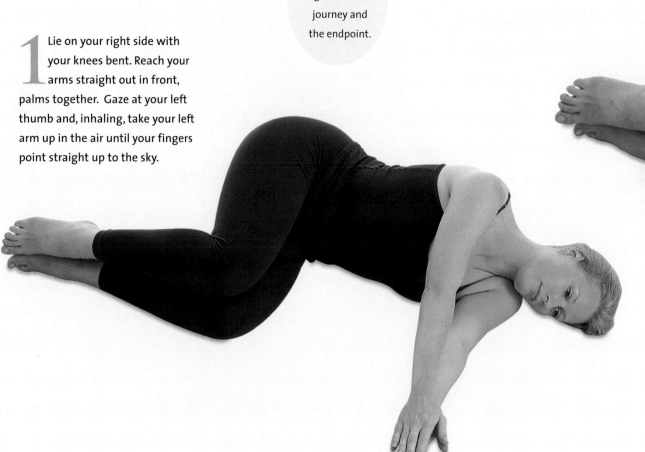

2 Exhale as you take your left arm towards the floor behind you. If you are flexible in the shoulders, the back of your hand may go all the way to the floor. On your next inhalation, bring your arm back up to halfway, still following its path with your eyes. Check you are not slumping into your left shoulder, but reaching away with your whole arm. Exhale it down to join the palms together.

Continue for six more rounds. As your breath is slow and constant, so is your rate of movement. Time the movement to follow the breath. Your fingers point skywards with the end of each inhalation. Your opening out and returning to base coincide with the end of the exhalation.

back of hand
resting on floor

knees bent

3 As you open out on the sixth round, let the back of your hand rest on the floor. Hold this position and take six deep breaths. Bring more of the left side of your back into contact with the floor as you deepen the twist in your waist. Reach your left arm away and feel your shoulders widen. This position gives a gentle opening of the chest. Don't rush on to the next inhalation between breaths, but allow it to arise naturally. As you lie quietly, each exhalation brings softening and release.

4 When you are ready to repeat on the right side, keep the arms spread apart, and inhale your legs up to centre and over to lie on your left side.

Cat pose

This exercise brings awareness and flexibility to the entire length of the spine. Channelling the breath into movement is centring and helps to keep the flow of the breath constant.

1 Start on all fours. Have your knees under your hips and your hands under your shoulders. Position the hands so both middle fingers stretch straight forward. Gaze at the floor between your hands in this neutral position.

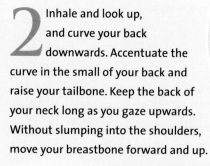

2 Inhale and look up, and curve your back downwards. Accentuate the curve in the small of your back and raise your tailbone. Keep the back of your neck long as you gaze upwards. Without slumping into the shoulders, move your breastbone forward and up.

TIP
Focus on a single vertebra for several rounds. Mentally go inside to feel how it works.

3 As you exhale, tuck your pelvis under, and round your back. Your upper back arches naturally in this way, but try to make the lower back curve in the same way. As you press each vertebra up to the sky, feel your shoulder blades spread apart and earth your palms by pressing them evenly to the floor. As you finish your exhalation, move your chin towards your breastbone.

Repeat ten more rounds, arching and curving in time to your breath. Maintain perfect awareness so that you curve deeper each time. To deepen it, walk the hands in 8cm (3in) to accentuate the curves.

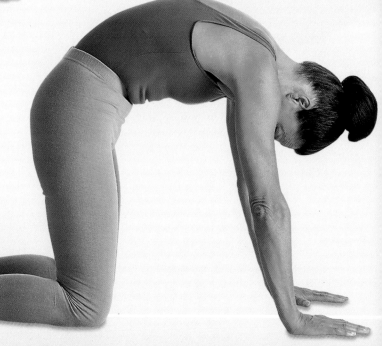

The **standing** poses

Our feet on the earth are often the base from which we operate. Standing poses give us the opportunity to explore our connection with the earth below our feet. They can teach us how to maintain a strong, stable base, while extending ourselves to soar skywards.

The lines created by the arms and legs are quite easily seen in the standing poses. Like strong rays of energy, they radiate out from the spine which feeds them. When the limbs are stretched to extend further away, a centred core through the spine is maintained.

The standing poses develop qualities of strength, focus and stability. They are poses in which you can relatively easily activate your muscles and joints and develop control over your body. Though the leg muscles work to keep you erect, don't allow this firmness in the muscles to freeze them, or make the breath irregular. Bring an element of softness and release to this firmness too.

In the wide stance poses, the further apart your feet, the greater the spinal extension, but balance becomes more difficult. The effort involved in balancing develops focus and concentration in the dance between stability and the extension of the self.

CAUTION
Avoid standing poses if you have acute asthma, colitis or cardiac problems.

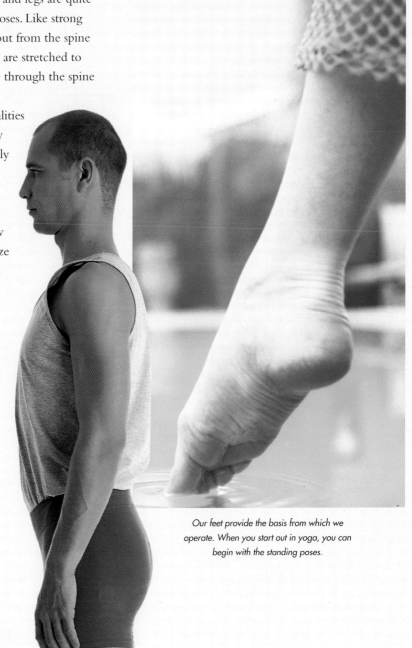

Our feet provide the basis from which we operate. When you start out in yoga, you can begin with the standing poses.

Standing tall

Achieving 'perfect posture' is not always a realistic goal. Years of stress and trauma have embedded themselves in the muscles and fascia, and compensatory ways of moving have been developed in response to injuries or pains. This results in protective patterns of holding the body being erected like physiological scaffolding. Don't despair if you have less than ideal alignment: few of us do. For change to occur, your first step has been to become aware of the irregularities. The next step is regular practice with attention both to alignment and undoing muscular tension, and yoga can help to balance the body.

The vertebral column has four curves. When a baby is born its whole spine is a convex 'C' shape. When the infant starts to raise its head the inward (concave) curve of the cervical vertebrae of its neck is formed. On sitting upright, the concave curve in its lower back (lumbar region) develops. The fourth curve is at the base of the spine, where the sacrum and tailbone (coccyx) maintain their original convex shape.

These curves act protectively as a kind of shock absorber. Although we often talk about a 'straight back', we don't actually mean one straight line. Rather, a healthy spine will have a balance between these four curves, with no part too flat or too rounded.

An exaggerated rounding of the thoracic region (upper back) is known as a kyphosis. Lordosis is an increased concavity in the lumbar region. Scoliosis is when the spine curves into a 'C' or 'S' shape and is noticeable from behind, not side on.

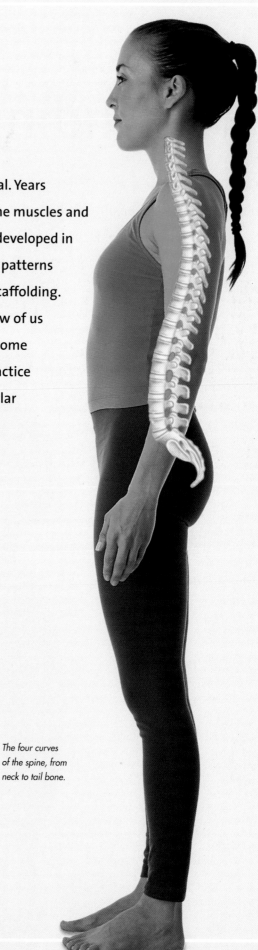

The four curves of the spine, from neck to tail bone.

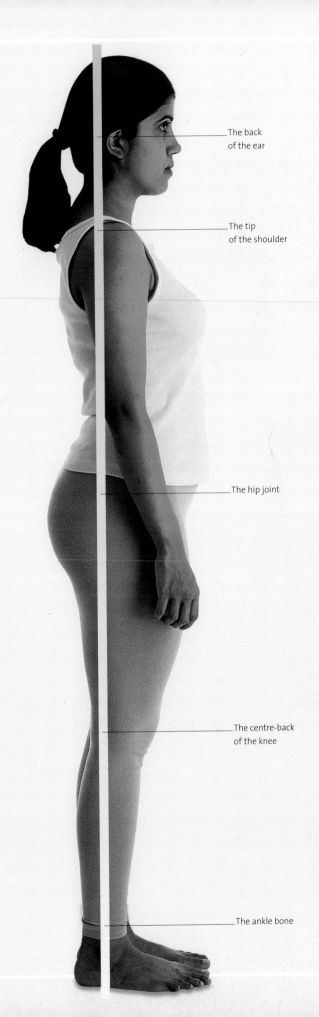

The back
of the ear

The tip
of the shoulder

The hip joint

The centre-back
of the knee

The ankle bone

sk a friend to help assess your posture. Dangle a
weighted cord from the side of your head to
your ankle so it lines up with the back of
your ear. Make a note of which 'landmarks' it passes
through on the way to the floor. In an ideal posture,
it will pass through the back of your ear, the tip of
your shoulder, the centre of your hip joint, the
centre-back of your knee and the back edge of your
anklebone.

If your plumbline doesn't follow these points,
keep in mind that often the disparity doesn't
originate from the obvious area, but from lower
down. Our base is from the ground up. Irregularities
in the feet (such as flattened arches, pigeon-toed or
turned out feet) will change the working of the
knees. Any problem in the knees (an injury, or
hyperextended 'pushed back' knees, for example) will
creep up to alter the way the hips work. Any foot,
knee or hip problem can potentially affect the back
and neck. Commonly, a lower back problem can, over
time, spread to become a neck complaint.

*In an ideal posture,
a plumbline would pass
through the body points
shown here.*

Samasthiti Equal pose

Begin and end each of the standing poses with this stable, centred pose. Practise Samasthiti whenever you are standing throughout the day.

1 Stand with your feet together or slightly apart, whichever feels most comfortable. Take your awareness to your soles and the distribution of weight between them. Do you have more weight on one foot than the other?

2 If you can balance, close your eyes. Slowly rock your weight from side to side, moving through the centre point of your feet. Now lean forwards and back slowly several times. Finally rest, centred. Bring an element of softness to your feet, so they feel as though they widen outwards.

3 While your feet ground downwards, move your awareness to your legs and get a sense of extending up towards the sky, starting at the ankle joints.

4 Expand your awareness to your torso. Let your pelvis be in a neutral position, neither tilted forward, nor back. (For more information, see Exploration: the role of the hips in forward bends, page 44.)

5 Exhale tension out of the spine so it is released to grow taller. Your abdomen moves in and out in time with your slow, rhythmic breath.

6 If you tend to round your back and 'collapse' in your chest area, lift your breastbone gently towards the chin. Make it subtle, so your floating ribs don't jut out. If you carry your chest expanded to the extent that you bring tension into your lower back, soften it and let go.

7 Drop your shoulders and let them hang relaxed. Aim for a feeling of width between the tips of your shoulders. Let your arms hang, with your fingers naturally curled slightly.

8 With your shoulders released, you will feel that your neck can extend up. The head is heavy but sometimes part of this weight is psychological! Let this unnecessary weight fly off so your head balances in a light, balloon-like way, on the top of your neck. Take slow, deep, steady breaths in this pose.

TIP

Rise up on tiptoes and breathe steadily for five breaths. Gaze at a fixed point exactly at eye level. Keep your eyes and head at this same height as you very slowly lower the heels to the floor. Feel how tall you are now!

Parsvakonasana
Side angle stretch

This pose gives a great stretch along the whole side of your body. If your head feels uncomfortable looking up in this pose, or the other standing poses, then look straight ahead.

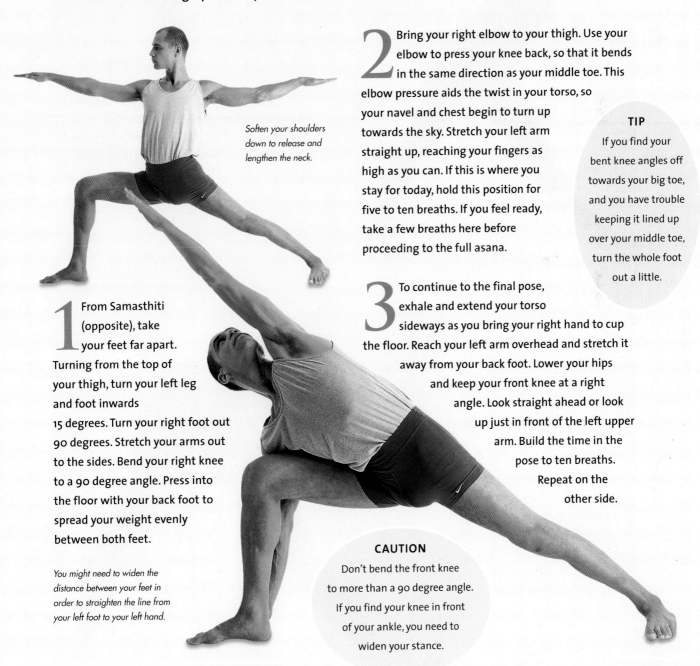

Soften your shoulders down to release and lengthen the neck.

1 From Samasthiti (opposite), take your feet far apart. Turning from the top of your thigh, turn your left leg and foot inwards 15 degrees. Turn your right foot out 90 degrees. Stretch your arms out to the sides. Bend your right knee to a 90 degree angle. Press into the floor with your back foot to spread your weight evenly between both feet.

You might need to widen the distance between your feet in order to straighten the line from your left foot to your left hand.

2 Bring your right elbow to your thigh. Use your elbow to press your knee back, so that it bends in the same direction as your middle toe. This elbow pressure aids the twist in your torso, so your navel and chest begin to turn up towards the sky. Stretch your left arm straight up, reaching your fingers as high as you can. If this is where you stay for today, hold this position for five to ten breaths. If you feel ready, take a few breaths here before proceeding to the full asana.

3 To continue to the final pose, exhale and extend your torso sideways as you bring your right hand to cup the floor. Reach your left arm overhead and stretch it away from your back foot. Lower your hips and keep your front knee at a right angle. Look straight ahead or look up just in front of the left upper arm. Build the time in the pose to ten breaths. Repeat on the other side.

TIP
If you find your bent knee angles off towards your big toe, and you have trouble keeping it lined up over your middle toe, turn the whole foot out a little.

CAUTION
Don't bend the front knee to more than a 90 degree angle. If you find your knee in front of your ankle, you need to widen your stance.

Trikonasana **Triangle pose**

This pose strengthens the legs and ankles, opens the hips and gives the trunk a strong side stretch.

Lengthen from the top of the thigh to the fingertips before you lower the arm.

Reach the fingertips to the sky

3 Keep the back of your neck long and look straight ahead, or tuck your chin slightly in and turn your head and gaze at your left thumb.

4 The hip bones, perineum, shoulders and hands should be on the same line as your feet. If you find your hips are back and your shoulders are forward of this line, then bring the supporting hand higher up your leg. Hold for five to ten breaths and then repeat on the left side.

TIP
In these wide stance standing poses, line up your feet so that the heel of your front foot bisects the centre of your back foot.

1 From Samasthiti (see page 22), jump or step the feet to twice hip-width apart. Turning from the thighs, turn the left foot in 15 degrees and the right foot out 90 degrees. Keep the knees facing the same direction as the toes. Put your hands on your hips to check your hips are the same height. Adjust if necessary.

2 Stretch the arms out to the sides. Exhale and bend from the top of the right thigh; extend your torso and right arm to the right. Feel the right side of your trunk growing longer before putting your right hand on to your thigh or shin. Bring your left arm into the air, following the line of your right arm.

Keep the top hip well back so it stays in line over the bottom hip.

Don't collapse the arches of the feet

Virabhadrasana 1 **Warrior 1**

This courageous pose, named after the powerful hero
Virabhadra, gathers strength from its solid base for
the triumphant lifted chest and raised arms.

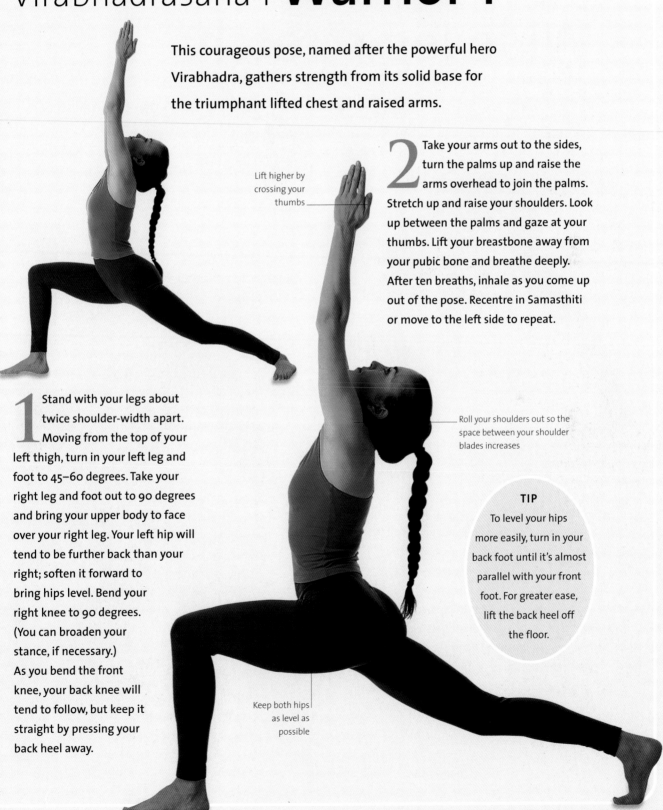

Lift higher by
crossing your
thumbs

2 Take your arms out to the sides,
turn the palms up and raise the
arms overhead to join the palms.
Stretch up and raise your shoulders. Look
up between the palms and gaze at your
thumbs. Lift your breastbone away from
your pubic bone and breathe deeply.
After ten breaths, inhale as you come up
out of the pose. Recentre in Samasthiti
or move to the left side to repeat.

Roll your shoulders out so the
space between your shoulder
blades increases

TIP
To level your hips
more easily, turn in your
back foot until it's almost
parallel with your front
foot. For greater ease,
lift the back heel off
the floor.

1 Stand with your legs about
twice shoulder-width apart.
Moving from the top of your
left thigh, turn in your left leg and
foot to 45–60 degrees. Take your
right leg and foot out to 90 degrees
and bring your upper body to face
over your right leg. Your left hip will
tend to be further back than your
right; soften it forward to
bring hips level. Bend your
right knee to 90 degrees.
(You can broaden your
stance, if necessary.)
As you bend the front
knee, your back knee will
tend to follow, but keep it
straight by pressing your
back heel away.

Keep both hips
as level as
possible

Prasarita padottanasana
Wide leg stretch

In the flowing, twisting action, use your breath as the starting point. Rather than adjusting your breath to follow your movement, time your movement to follow your breath.

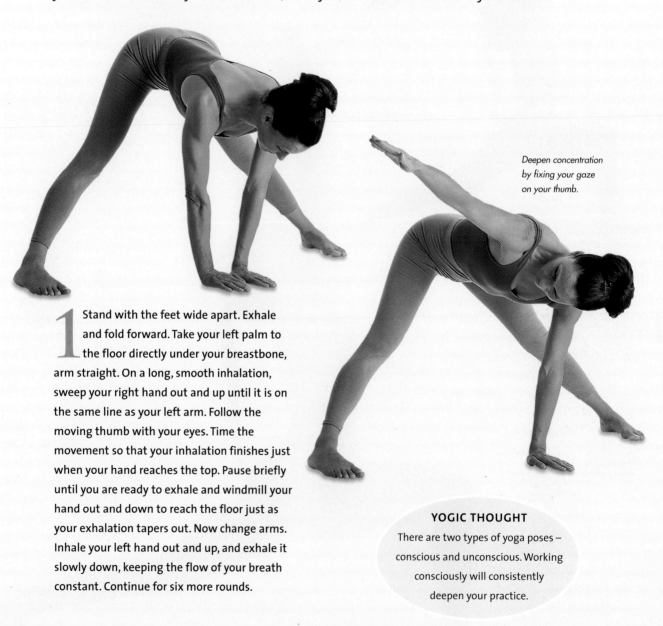

Deepen concentration by fixing your gaze on your thumb.

1 Stand with the feet wide apart. Exhale and fold forward. Take your left palm to the floor directly under your breastbone, arm straight. On a long, smooth inhalation, sweep your right hand out and up until it is on the same line as your left arm. Follow the moving thumb with your eyes. Time the movement so that your inhalation finishes just when your hand reaches the top. Pause briefly until you are ready to exhale and windmill your hand out and down to reach the floor just as your exhalation tapers out. Now change arms. Inhale your left hand out and up, and exhale it slowly down, keeping the flow of your breath constant. Continue for six more rounds.

YOGIC THOUGHT
There are two types of yoga poses – conscious and unconscious. Working consciously will consistently deepen your practice.

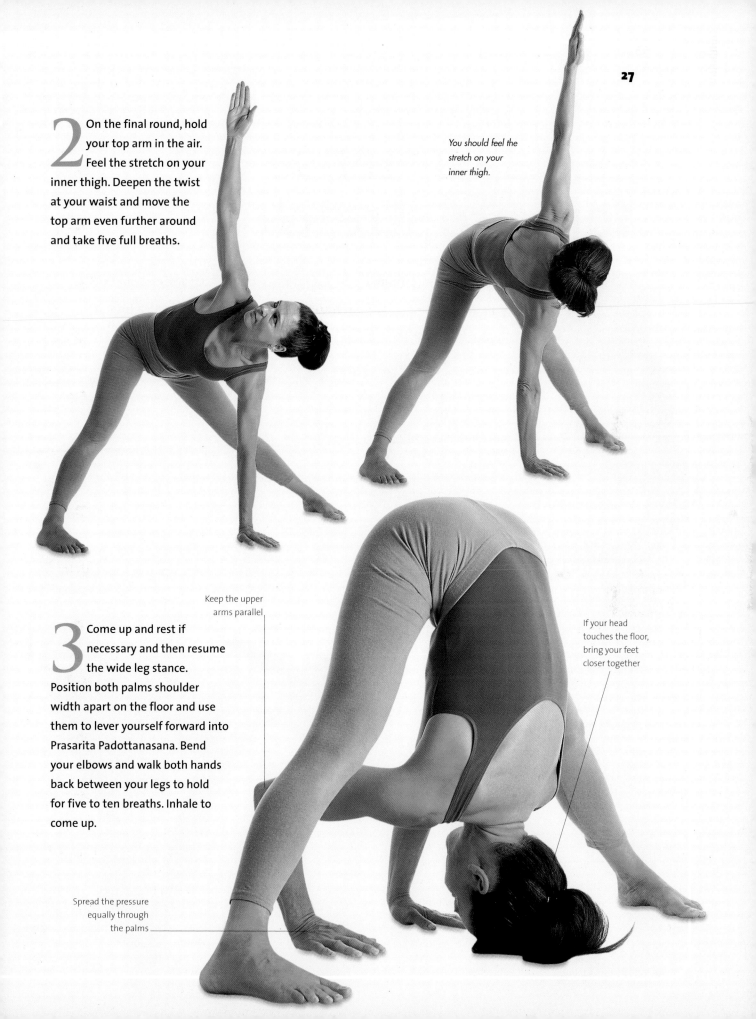

2 On the final round, hold your top arm in the air. Feel the stretch on your inner thigh. Deepen the twist at your waist and move the top arm even further around and take five full breaths.

You should feel the stretch on your inner thigh.

Keep the upper arms parallel

3 Come up and rest if necessary and then resume the wide leg stance. Position both palms shoulder width apart on the floor and use them to lever yourself forward into Prasarita Padottanasana. Bend your elbows and walk both hands back between your legs to hold for five to ten breaths. Inhale to come up.

If your head touches the floor, bring your feet closer together

Spread the pressure equally through the palms

Uttanasana **Intense forward stretch**

As the translation of the Sanskrit implies, this is a strong forward bend. However, it can also be used more passively to rest, offering a lesson in 'undoing' rather than 'doing'.

1 Stand with your feet hip width apart. Place your hands on your hips and, inhaling, squeeze your elbows closer together behind. Expand your chest so you get a sense of the breastbone moving up and away from the pubic bone. Exhale and, hinging at the hips, fold your torso over your legs. If your hamstrings are tight, bend your knees to access the hinging action of the hips before folding forward.

2 Exhale and fold forwards (see below). With knees bent or straight, maintain your fullest possible forward fold. As your hands grasp, ease your elbows to the sides. Being upside down, your shoulders will tend to fall towards the floor. Slide shoulder blades towards your hips to unhunch them.

3 Grasp your calves or ankles or loop your big toes with your fingers (see right, top). Straighten your arms, look up and, for the duration of several inhalations, increase the distance between your pubic bone and the base of your throat.

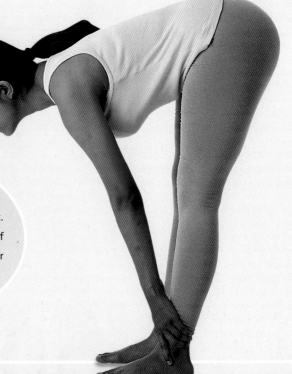

TIP
Working the feet correctly in the standing poses helps retrain flat feet. Anchor your inner heel and mound of your big toe and, without rolling your ankles out, lift your arches. so they are like rainbows.

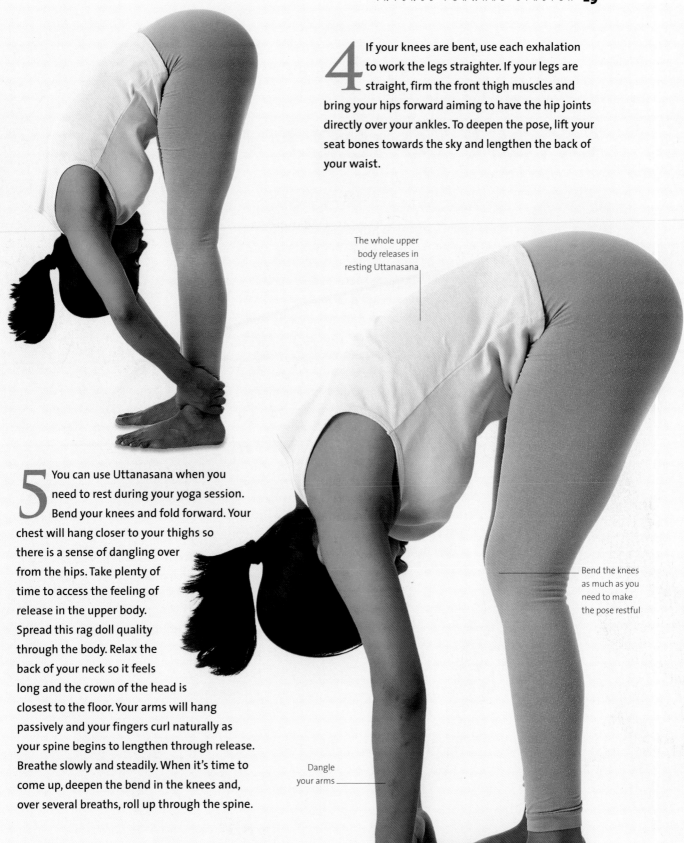

4 If your knees are bent, use each exhalation to work the legs straighter. If your legs are straight, firm the front thigh muscles and bring your hips forward aiming to have the hip joints directly over your ankles. To deepen the pose, lift your seat bones towards the sky and lengthen the back of your waist.

The whole upper body releases in resting Uttanasana

Bend the knees as much as you need to make the pose restful

5 You can use Uttanasana when you need to rest during your yoga session. Bend your knees and fold forward. Your chest will hang closer to your thighs so there is a sense of dangling over from the hips. Take plenty of time to access the feeling of release in the upper body. Spread this rag doll quality through the body. Relax the back of your neck so it feels long and the crown of the head is closest to the floor. Your arms will hang passively and your fingers curl naturally as your spine begins to lengthen through release. Breathe slowly and steadily. When it's time to come up, deepen the bend in the knees and, over several breaths, roll up through the spine.

Dangle your arms

Parsvottanasana
Chest to leg extension

This pose will help stretch not only legs and chest but the whole body.

1 From Samasthiti (see page 22), take your feet to twice shoulder width apart. Turn your left knee and foot in 60 degrees. Turn your right thigh, knee and foot out 90 degrees. Open your left groin, so that your upper body can face more over the right leg. Your left hip can then move forwards to align with your right and you can better line up your breastbone with the inside of your right thigh.

2 Take the backs of your hands as high as possible between your shoulder blades. Roll the shoulders and elbows back as you press your palms together into prayer pose. If your shoulders are tight, try holding your wrists behind your back. As a preparation for folding forward, inhale, lift your chest and look up.

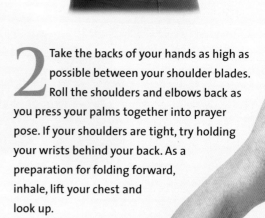

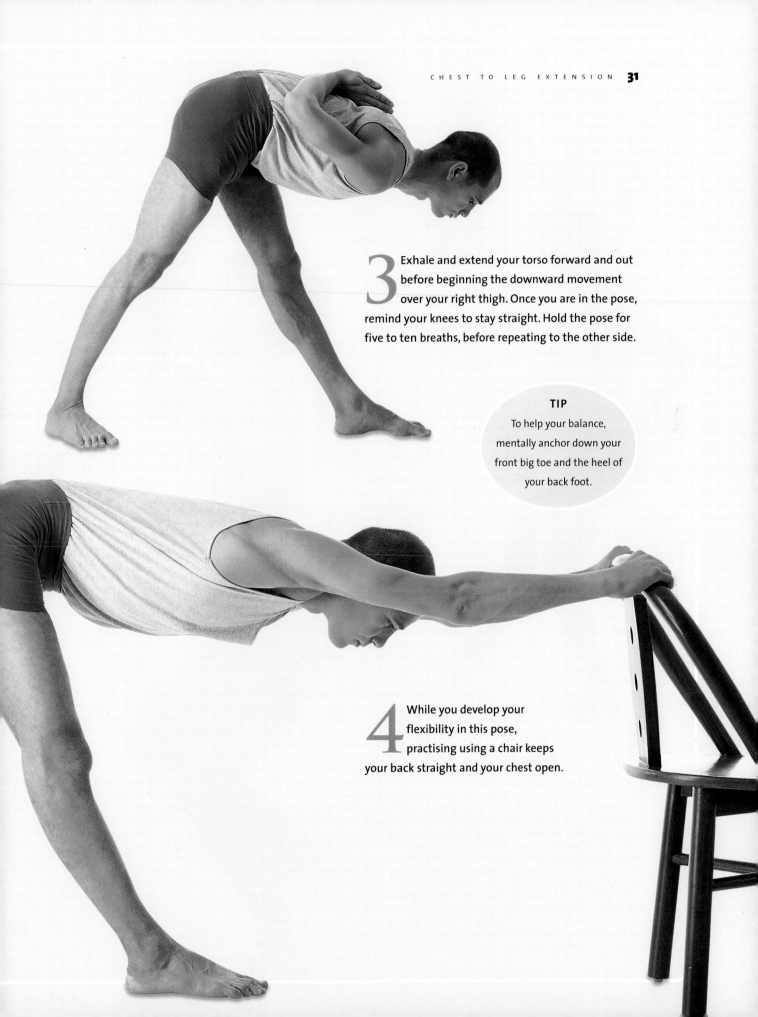

3 Exhale and extend your torso forward and out before beginning the downward movement over your right thigh. Once you are in the pose, remind your knees to stay straight. Hold the pose for five to ten breaths, before repeating to the other side.

TIP
To help your balance, mentally anchor down your front big toe and the heel of your back foot.

4 While you develop your flexibility in this pose, practising using a chair keeps your back straight and your chest open.

Garudasana **Eagle pose**

Grounding and concentration are keys to balance poses such as this.

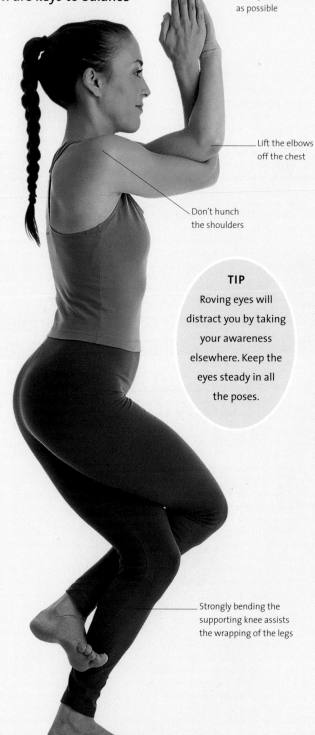

Bring both sets of fingertips as level as possible

Lift the elbows off the chest

Don't hunch the shoulders

Strongly bending the supporting knee assists the wrapping of the legs

1 From Samasthiti (see page 22), focus your gaze on a fixed point level with your eyes. Tune into the connection between the soles of your feet and the earth. Focus this awareness on your right foot and bend the left knee. Bend your right supporting leg strongly, and use the momentum to take your right leg around your left.

TIP
Roving eyes will distract you by taking your awareness elsewhere. Keep the eyes steady in all the poses.

2 Now wrap your arms by crossing your elbows left over right and bring the palms to face each other. The fingers of your right hand should be high up towards those of your right. You will be able to breathe into the chest more fully if you raise the elbows to shoulder level. If this is easy for you, roll your shoulders back and down. To stretch your shoulders further, ease your forearms forwards so your thumbs move away from your nose. Maintain the pose for ten breaths, before unwrapping, regrounding and repeating on the opposite side.

Back bends

Back bends stretch the abdominal area, increasing the blood supply to the kidneys, pancreas and reproductive system. By opening the solar plexus and stimulating what yogis call the solar nerve, which physiologically relates to the sympathetic nervous system, they are extremely invigorating. Back bends develop willpower and determination and cause inertia and laziness to dissipate.

Back bends are all-involving and exhilarating. In a strong back bend, it seems there is no space left for new thoughts to arise. It's hard to think about anything else, so they are good for freeing yourself from distracting thoughts. They involve the fiery digestive energies and have a warming effect on the body. If you try doing a few back bends in a cold room, you will soon feel warm inside.

Back bends open and lift the heart centre at the chest. They create space for joy to reside in the body.

While you intimately know the front of your body, probably the best view you have had of your back is second-hand, through the reflection of a mirror. As we naturally tend to place more emphasis on the things we see, back bends allow you to practise spreading awareness in your body to other parts.

Bending backwards is a step into the unknown. While we often bend forwards in our day to day lives, we rarely bend backwards. Conquer the fear of the unfamiliar, maintain faith and bend towards the unknown.

Always warm up with standing postures before beginning back bends, and to follow them with some twists and forward bends to release your back and cool the system. Those with hypertension should work with an experienced teacher.

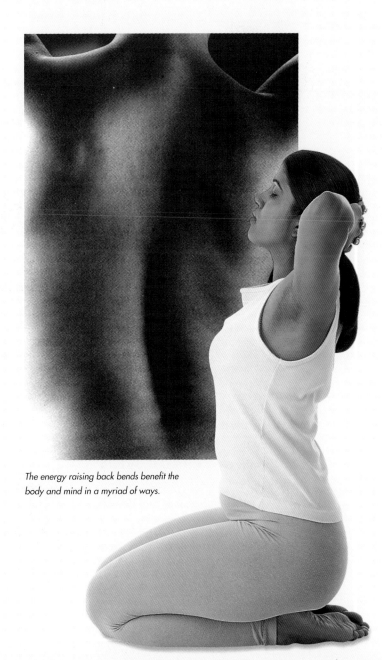

The energy raising back bends benefit the body and mind in a myriad of ways.

Exploration
Preparations for back bending

Rehearse the isolated movements for bending backwards before you unite them in the back bending asanas.

1 Sit on your heels and interlace your fingers behind your head, keeping your shoulders relaxed. As you inhale open your elbows out to the side and back. If you keep your head well supported with your hands, you can keep the back of your neck long as you look up. This feeling of the neck staying long is what you are aiming for in back bends such as the cobra and locust poses.

2 Exhale and slowly bring your elbows closer together in front of you, as you take your chin towards your breastbone. Don't press the head down with your hands. Move between these two positions ten times. With each inhalation, focus on the curving of your upper back and neck. Feel the expansion in your ribs. Let each exhalation be long and slow as you soften your upper body.

You will experience a feeling of the back being 'lengthened'.

3 Now come up to a kneeling position. Interlace your fingers behind you, so your knuckles rest on either side of the spine below the shoulder blades. Take time to anchor down through the knees. Lengthen your front thighs by tucking your tailbone under and opening your groin. On an inhalation, press your hands into your back, squeeze your elbows towards each other and lift your breastbone as you bend backwards. Maintain the long neck from the first exercise and don't take your neck back beyond its comfort level.

4 Press your knuckles into the sides of your spine and, as your chest lifts and opens, get a feeling of lifting the vertebrae up and over them. While you will naturally feel long in the front, maintain the length in the back of your body as much as possible. Remember this feeling of the long back so you can reproduce it in each back bending asana.

5 As you exhale relax your shoulders down and your elbows forwards and come back to a neutral position. Complete ten more rounds.

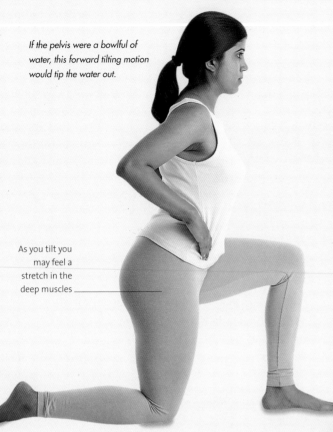

If the pelvis were a bowlful of water, this forward tilting motion would tip the water out.

As you tilt you may feel a stretch in the deep muscles

9 This tipping back action is good practice for safe back bending. Back bends start from the very base of the spine, not the lumbar region. The tailbone needs to lengthen down towards the ground. This initial flattening out of the lower back lengthens the vertebrae away from each other, as preparation for a long, deep curve.

10 Keep your chest and shoulders steady as you inhale while tipping forwards and exhale while tipping backwards. Allow plenty of time to begin to isolate this movement.

6 Kneel on your right knee and bend your left leg in front. Place your hands on your hipbones with your thumbs facing back and your fingers forwards.

7 Imagine your pelvis is a container full of water and you want to pour the water out slowly. First, tilt your pelvis forwards so that you feel your fingers move down and your thumbs move up as if you were pouring the water out the front.

8 Now tip your pelvis back the other way, as if you were pouring water behind you. Your fingers raise up and the curve in your lower back flattens out. Do it slowly and you will feel a deep stretch in the front of the left thigh.

The fingers on the iliac crest will rise as the forward tilt is reversed

Reverse the tilt so the lower back flattens

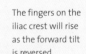

Bhujangasana **Cobra pose**

As you form the shape of a cobra, it's like rising up to meet an obstacle in your path.

1 Lie on your front with your feet together and your forehead touching the floor. Place your palms on the floor so your fingertips are level with the tips of the shoulders, and your elbows are in the air. Roll your shoulders back and down away from your ears, so they move towards your hips. Squeeze your elbows towards each other and feel the length in the back of the neck.

2 Slightly tilt your pelvis by pressing your pubic bone to the floor. When you do this, you can reach your toes back further and the back of your waist lengthens.

3 Curl your head and shoulders up as far as you can without taking weight on your hands. Hold this position to find out which back muscles need to work. Now press the hands to the floor as you curve up higher, shoulders down and neck long. Your elbows stay deeply bent and your hips stay on the floor. Hold three repetitions for ten breaths. When you inhale deeply, your abdominal organs are massaged as your abdomen presses on the floor.

TIP
From your starting position, lift one leg at a time and stretch it back. Observe how this gives more length in the lower back.

4 Extend the inner body as you 'pump' the breastbone forward and up on each inhalation. Lower the shoulders and the outer body on each exhalation to lengthen the inner body.

5 Make a pillow with your hands and rest with your head to alternate sides between each repetition.

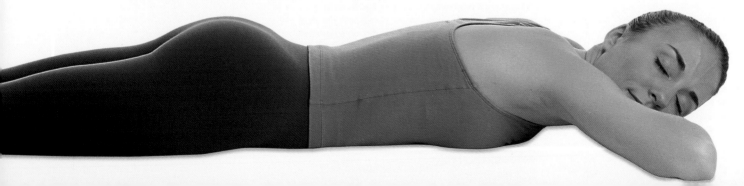

Salabhasana **Locust pose**

This pose is strengthening for the back and opening for the chest. Its action on the back is best if you keep your ankles together.

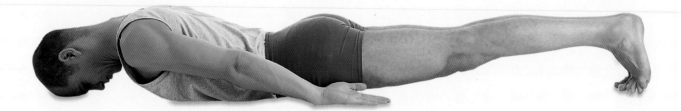

1 Lie on your front with your feet together and your forehead on the floor, arms by your side. Tuck your toes under, stretch your heels away and lift up the knees. Firm your thighs and keep both legs straight. Move your tailbone towards your feet and stretch both heels back to elongate the back.

2 Now flick your toes away and lift your straight legs up in the air. Lift your arms and curl your head and chest up off the floor. Lengthen the crown of your head and your tailbone away from each other. Your back bend will deepen as you press both shoulders away from your ears and reach your fingers towards the toes. Build to hold three repetitions for ten breaths each. Between repetitions, relax down and turn your head to one side and observe your breathing as it returns to normal.

CAUTION

If you suffer from back problems, keep your chest on the floor and lift one leg at a time, stretching it well back. Then keep your feet well anchored to the floor and lift only your upper body and arms.

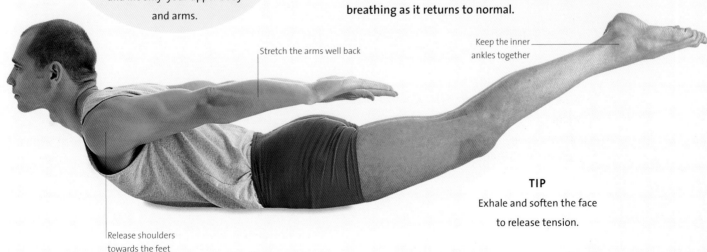

Stretch the arms well back

Keep the inner ankles together

Release shoulders towards the feet

TIP
Exhale and soften the face to release tension.

Setu Bandhasana **Bridge pose**

As you open your chest, expand your heart centre in this pose.

1 Lie on your back with the knees bent up. Place your feet 15cm (6in) away from your buttocks and have them as wide as your hipbones.

TIP

Don't let your knees splay apart – keep them only as wide as your hips.

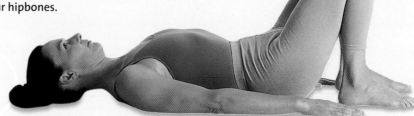

2 Begin by tilting your pelvis slightly so your buttocks move off the ground. Your lower, middle and upper back will still be connected to the floor. Take several breaths in this position.

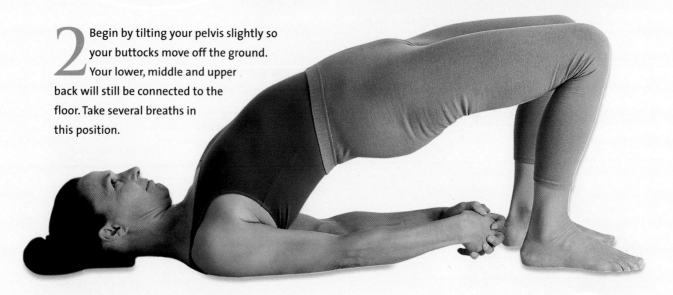

3 Now, while constantly stretching your knees away, slowly lift your hips higher. With your hips raised up, tuck your shoulders under one by one. Squeeze the shoulder blades in together and shift more weight onto the tips of the shoulders. If your elbows can straighten, interlace your fingers and press them down to lift and open the chest.

4 A bridge reaches in both directions to the river banks. While the breastbone moves towards your chin, the tailbone moves towards the knees. After holding five to ten breaths come down and rest. Repeat twice more.

YOGIC THOUGHT

Have patience as you approach each new edge in a pose. Respect the body and wait for it to let you in.

Matsyasana Fish pose

Matsyasana hyperextends the neck. It is excellent after both the Sarvangasana (page 65) and Halasana (page 67) where the neck is strongly flexed.

1 Lying on your back, take your hands, palms down, under your thighs. Reach your fingertips as far as you can towards the backs of the knees.

TIP
Bring your awareness to the back of the body. Develop the sensitivity of the skin on the back as it thins out in each back bend.

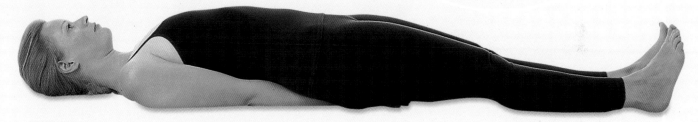

2 Inhale and come up so you are resting on your elbows. Squeeze your shoulder blades in together, then exhale and release the crown of your head lightly to the floor. Expand your chest and draw each inhalation deeper. In Matsyasana, only about 10 per cent of your weight is on the crown of the head, and the rest is supported by the elbows and lower body. Hold for five to ten breaths.

Open the chest with each inhalation

Lower the crown of the head lightly to the floor

The elbows support most of the weight of the upper body

3 To come up, inhale strongly as you move the weight forward onto your elbows and lift your head. Bring your chin to your chest as you lower down to rest on your back. Release your neck by gently turning your head to take alternate ears to the floor.

Chakrasana **Wheel pose**

Recharge with this demanding, but highly energising pose.

1 Lie on your back, with your knees bent and your feet 20cm (8in) from your buttocks. Place your hands near the shoulders, fingers pointing in the direction of the hips. Take some time to breathe while anchoring down through your heels.

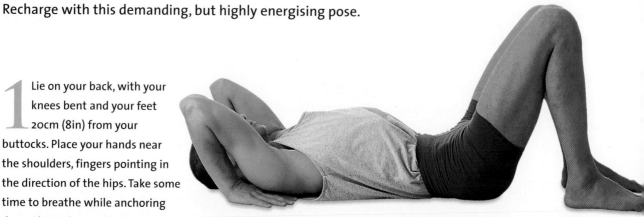

2 Lift your hips up, then inhale and lift up on to the crown of your head. Breathe here as you mentally prepare to lift all the way up. Pressurise the palms, inhale and straighten the arms to lift into the full position.

CAUTION

This pose is not advisable in cases of slipped disc, hernia, heart problems, high blood pressure, during menstruation, pregnancy or in the post-natal period.

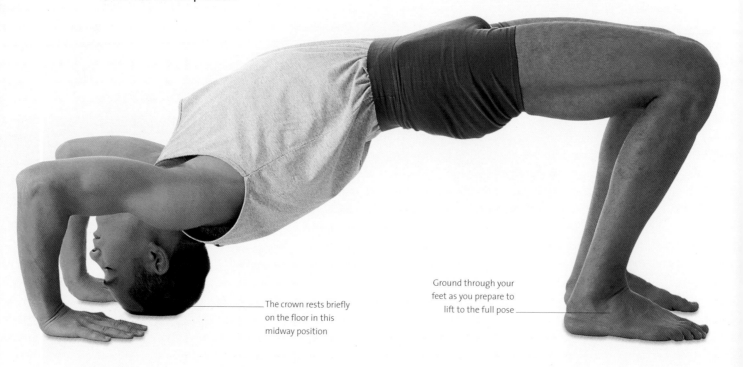

The crown rests briefly on the floor in this midway position

Ground through your feet as you prepare to lift to the full pose

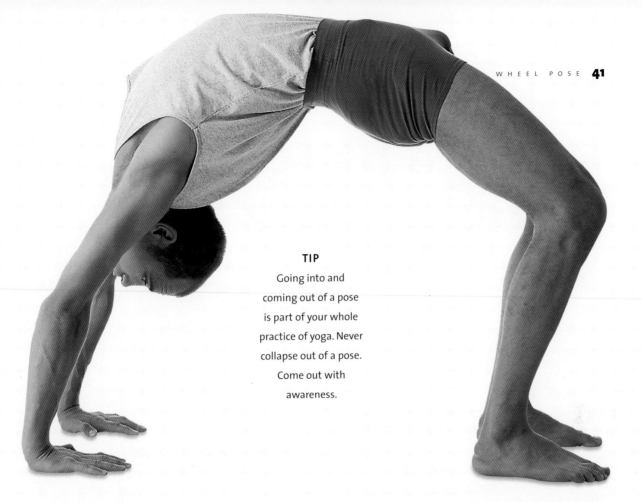

TIP
Going into and
coming out of a pose
is part of your whole
practice of yoga. Never
collapse out of a pose.
Come out with
awareness.

3 Now you are up, make a few adjustments. In the effort of coming up, your toes will tend to turn out and your knees move apart. Bring your feet back to parallel, then reposition your knees over your feet.

4 While in the classic pose the heels are on the ground, come on to your tiptoes until you can straighten the arms. Keep the heels up if you need to build the flexibility to prevent compressing your lower back when the heels are lowered. Now visualise a circle of energy moving between the hands and the toes. Lift and move your sacrum around this wheel towards your knees. Push up into the fronts of your thighs and open your groin more. Expand the chest.

5 Hold and breathe for five to ten breaths. When you come down, tuck the chin in and lower down with control. Rest and feel the difference in your body and mind after doing this pose. Repeat twice more – it usually feels best of all the third time.

6 Ease out your back by hugging your knees into your chest and rocking slowly from side to side. The slower you rock, the nicer this massage feels.

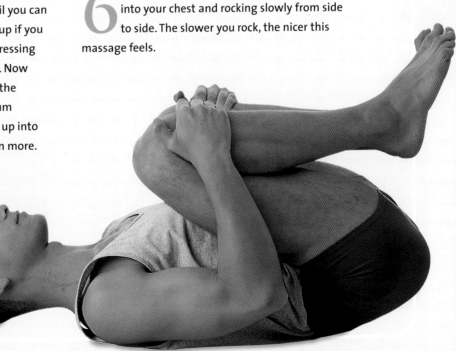

Forward bends and seated posture

After bending backwards, now fold the other way to stretch the whole back of the body and increase the vitality of the spine.

Forward bends aid digestion and general well-being by nourishing the abdominal organs. Bending forward stimulates the nerve ganglions of the parasympathetic nervous system in the pelvis. This nervous system is involved in resting the body, repairing the cells and restoring the body to health.

While bending backwards increases alertness, bending forwards promotes introspection and helps quieten the mind. Folding into yourself lets you access your intuitive self and become more self-aware. As a modified curling up action, forward bends feel safe and nurturing. For all the seated postures, take nourishment from the support by the earth.

Use forward bends when you are tired or after a hard day. Make them more restorative by stacking up pillows or bolsters to fold over and support your head by resting your forehead on one. This rests the frontal lobe of the brain and is calming and helps you to recentre.

Those suffering from a slipped disc need to keep some concavity in the back. Under the guidance of an experienced yoga teacher, a modified practice of forward bends can be built. Forward bends should be avoided in cases of severe depression.

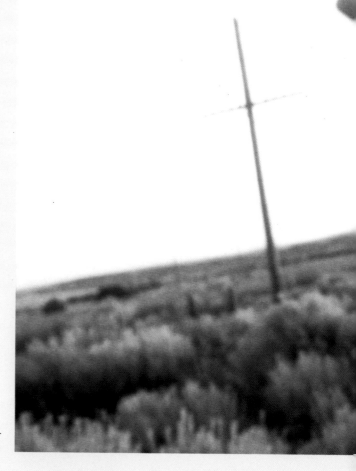

Forward bends and seated posture enhance your sense of well-being and help you to recentre.

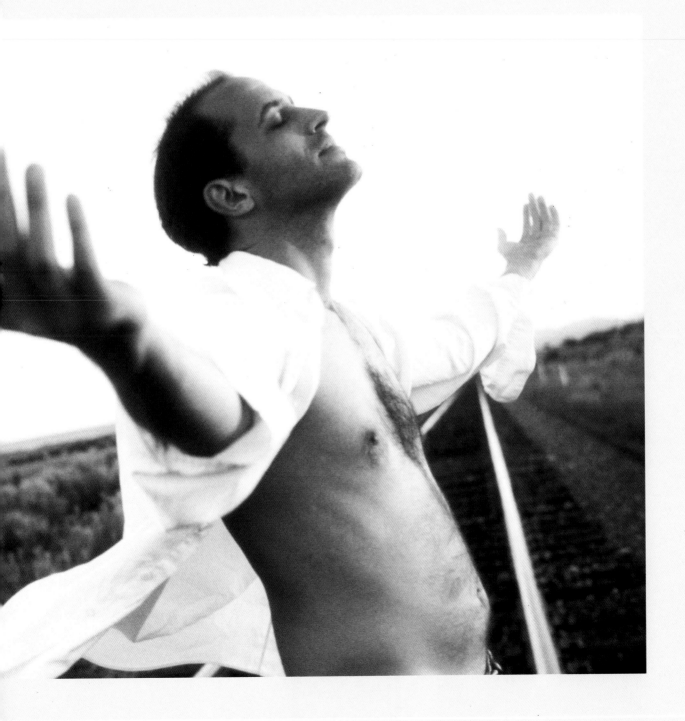

Exploration The role of the hips in forward bends

Isolate the hip movement for correct alignment in forward bends.

1 Sit on a chair and place your hands on your hipbones, fingers facing forwards. Rock the pelvis back so your thumbs move down and fingers tilt up. Your lower back will feel as though it flattens out on this upward tilting.

2 The key movement for forward bends follows. Tilt your pelvis forwards so your fingers move forward and down. The desired action comes from the hip joint. Your thighbones stay still and you are rotating the hip socket around the stationary head of the thighbone. Tilt the hips slowly back and forth. It may take a while for the movement to come. It is vital in forward bending to move the stretch to the back of the thighs and not overstretch the lower back.

3 A common mistake if this hip action comes with difficulty is to sway the chest back and forth, causing the floating ribs to jut out. In the correct action, the vertebral column stays quite straight; the chest and shoulders move only slightly.

A common mistake is to sway the chest back and forth

4 Once you have this feeling, refine this movement. Raise your seat 20cm (8in) from the floor by sitting on a small stool or firm cushions. Tilt back and forth, repeating the action of rotating your pelvis around the heads of the thigh bones. As you tilt forward, the crease at the top of your thighs will deepen and you may feel your seat bones jut out more behind you.

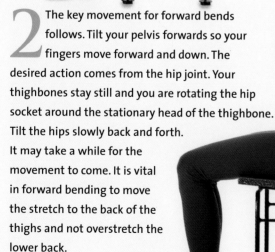

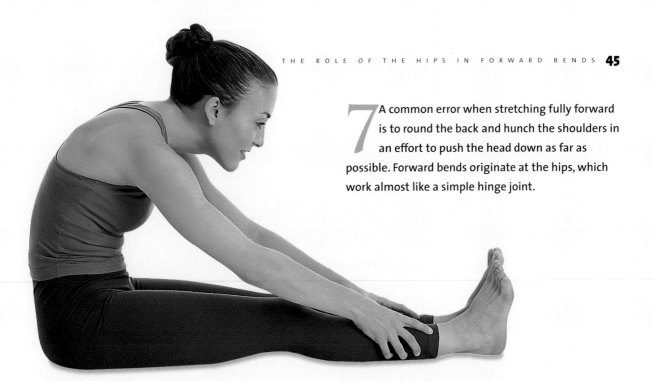

7 A common error when stretching fully forward is to round the back and hunch the shoulders in an effort to push the head down as far as possible. Forward bends originate at the hips, which work almost like a simple hinge joint.

5 For the third stage, sit on the floor and practise this same movement. If, from this lower position, you can't access it, bend your knees. It helps if you can feel your sit bones on the floor, so use your hands to move your buttock flesh back and out to the sides.

6 If it feels very difficult, as if your hips are frozen, it could be a sign of tight hamstrings. If your pelvis tilts backwards when you sit up straight, and your stomach muscles have to work strongly just to keep you upright, then modify your starting position. Lift your seat with a cushion, and bend your knees if necessary.

8 As you hinge forwards, keep your back straight so that your navel will reach your thighs before your chest reaches your knees. Only then will your nose come to your shins. Remind yourself of this during every forward bend, and think of forward folding rather than bending.

Keep the back flat, not curved

Keep the chest open as you fold forwards

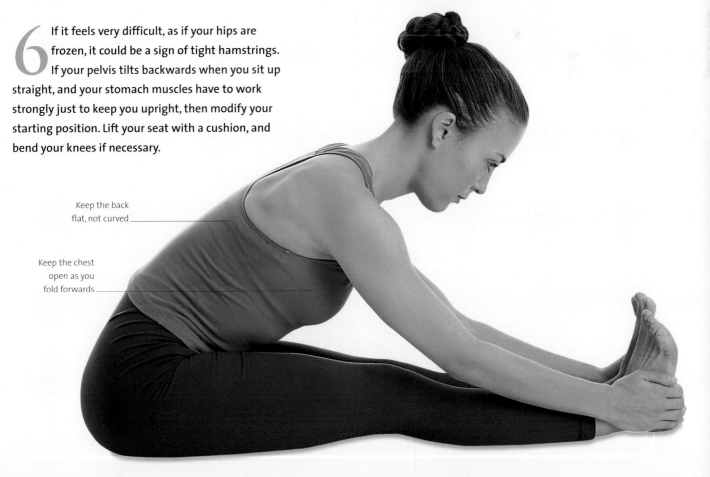

Adho Mukha Svanasana
Downward-facing dog

This is an excellent pose for stretching and strengthening the whole body. Though it may not feel like it at first, with practice it can become very restful.

TIP

Use downward-facing dog as a link between other postures in your practice.

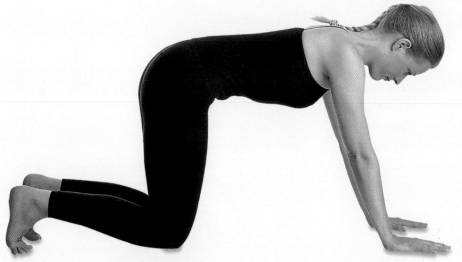

1 Begin on all fours. Have your knees and feet hip width apart. Walk your hands forwards 15cm (6in) so they are in front of, not directly below, your shoulders. To protect your wrists, check that your middle fingers are facing straight forwards. Get a sense of your hands pressing into the earth. Feel how your weight is distributed on the palms. Aim for an even spread from the base of your hand right to your fingertips.

2 Tuck your toes under and lift your hips high until you are in an inverted V position. Bend your right knee and exhale as you stretch your left heel towards the floor. Change sides and allow the muscles on the back of your right leg to release. Working with the breath, warm your hamstrings by moving back and forth from right to left.

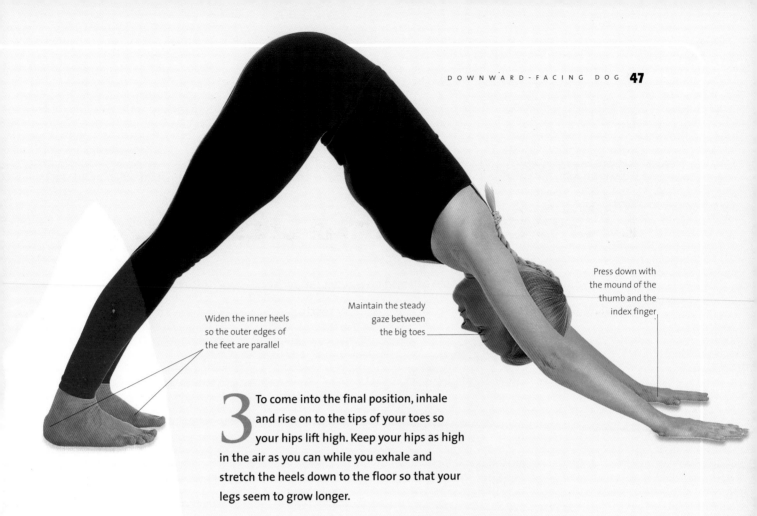

Press down with
the mound of the
thumb and the
index finger

Maintain the steady
gaze between
the big toes

Widen the inner heels
so the outer edges of
the feet are parallel

3 To come into the final position, inhale
and rise on to the tips of your toes so
your hips lift high. Keep your hips as high
in the air as you can while you exhale and
stretch the heels down to the floor so that your
legs seem to grow longer.

4 Widen the shoulder blades apart by rolling
your upper arms outwards. Aim for one
straight line from wrists to buttocks. Root the
mounds of your thumbs and index fingers to keep the
pressure evenly spread through your palms. In this
inverted position, the spine hangs down from the
hips. Get a sense of extension in your spine through
letting go, rather than using effort, to lengthen.
Maintain the downward-facing dog pose for five
to 15 steady breaths.

DEEPEN IT
Play with this pose by practising
the backwards and forwards pelvic tilt
(see page 44). It gives you the option of
increasing flexibility in the backs of the thighs
or stretching more into the lower back to
release tension there instead.

5 To rest after this pose,
bring your big toes
together, knees wide
apart, and rest your hips back
to your heels until the breath
has steadied.

Trianga Mukhaikapada Paschimottanasana
Three-limbed bend

Though it can feel awkward at first, due to its particular action on the hips, this pose is a good lead off for the seated forward bends.

TIP

Keep the ankle of the straight leg flexed and stretch the heel away in all the forward bends.

2 Before you think about going forward, it's useful to sit erect and breathe yourself taller for a short while. When you are ready, inhale as you bring your arms overhead, and exhale as you extend forward to grasp your calf, ankle or foot. Inhale, lift your chest and look up. Exhale, bend your elbows to the sides, and fold forward with a flat back and open chest. Hold for five to ten breaths before repeating on the other side.

3 To lessen tilting and to keep your spine straight, have a folded blanket under your bent leg side.

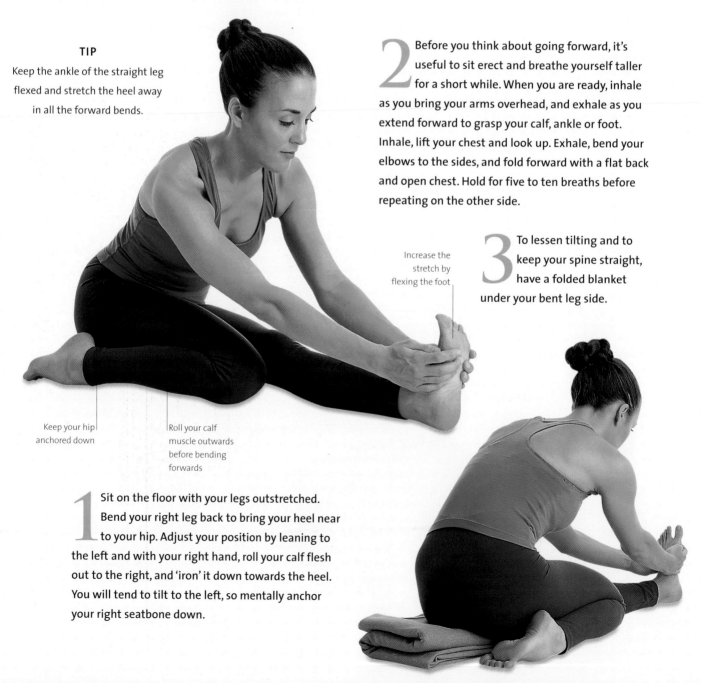

Increase the stretch by flexing the foot

Keep your hip anchored down

Roll your calf muscle outwards before bending forwards

1 Sit on the floor with your legs outstretched. Bend your right leg back to bring your heel near to your hip. Adjust your position by leaning to the left and with your right hand, roll your calf flesh out to the right, and 'iron' it down towards the heel. You will tend to tilt to the left, so mentally anchor your right seatbone down.

Janu Sirsasana Head beyond the knee pose

Make a big job less daunting by dividing it in half. Use this pose to prepare for Paschimottanasana (see overleaf), by stretching one leg at a time.

1 Sit with both legs straight in front of you. Bend your right leg out to the side so your heel is near your groin, and 3cm (1in) away from your left inner thigh. Don't let your toes slip under your thigh. Stretch your left heel away so that your knee and toes point straight up.

2 You will find this pose easier with a preparatory twist. Taking your left hand behind you and your right hand to the outer left knee, twist left for a few breaths.

3 Untwist slightly, and line up your breastbone so that it is over your left thigh. Inhale and lengthen up from your pubic bone to the base of your throat. Exhale and fold forwards. Hold your calf, side of the foot or left wrist around the foot. Use your arms to lever your torso deeper over your right thigh.

4 Sitting on a folded blanket allows you to fold a little deeper. Loop a belt around your foot to maintain correct alignment in the forward bends.

DEEPEN IT

Try a more advanced way of working to still the fluctuations in the body. If you hold a pose for ten breaths, use the first three to adjust and deepen it. For the remaining seven, hold still and open yourself to perceive and observe. You are moving neither from nor towards anything. Find the still point.

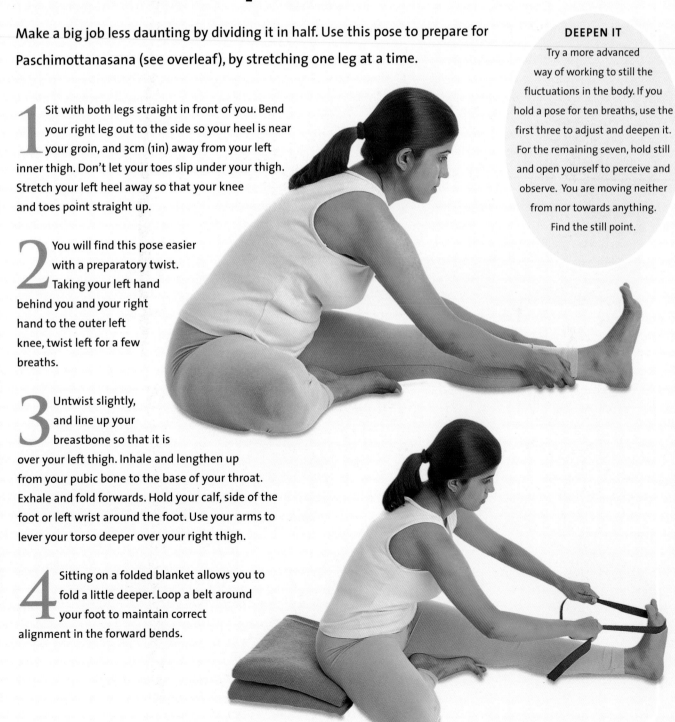

Paschimottanasana Stretch on the body's west side

Traditionally the west side of the body relates to the back of the body and the outer self. In this sequence, use visualisation as you fold into the east side – your inner self.

1 Sit quietly and think of some way you would like spring-clean your life. Perhaps you feel your life could be better with less aggression, hate or envy. Maybe you would like to remove a health problem, or feelings of doubt, indecision or laziness. Keep in mind the quality you decide on, inhale to bring your hands near your chest.

TIP

Yoga is not impulsive. Perform asanas slowly to become aware of your actions, reactions, intentions and thoughts. Leave time to receive feedback from your body between poses.

Exhale and sweep your hands down the front of your body.

2 Now, exhale and sweep your hands down the entire front of your body and out past your feet. Inhale as you bring your arms up in a wide arc and exhale as you push away what is unwanted, out of your body and out of your life. Repeat six more of these cleansing cycles, or as many as you feel necessary.

3 Now, pause and consider what you would like more of in your life. Would you feel better off with more compassion, enthusiasm, love, joy or humility in your life? Do you seek contentment, truth or wisdom?

Visualisation is an important step to creating a life as you want it.

4 This time reverse the flow. Start with your hands at your feet and draw your palms up close to your body as you sweep that desired quality into your life. Lean back, take your arms up in the air, exhale and reach forward. Inhale and sweep up again to continue welcoming that special quality. Repeat six more cycles, or more if you like.

5 Now prepare to hold the pose steady. Grasp your feet, ankles or calves. Inhale and lift the chest up so the front of the torso is long. Exhale to extend forward. In this folded position, your back is turned on what is unwelcome and you can gather that special quality into your world. Take long, slow breaths for 10 to 15 rounds.

Not concaving your chest will allow your heart centre to open

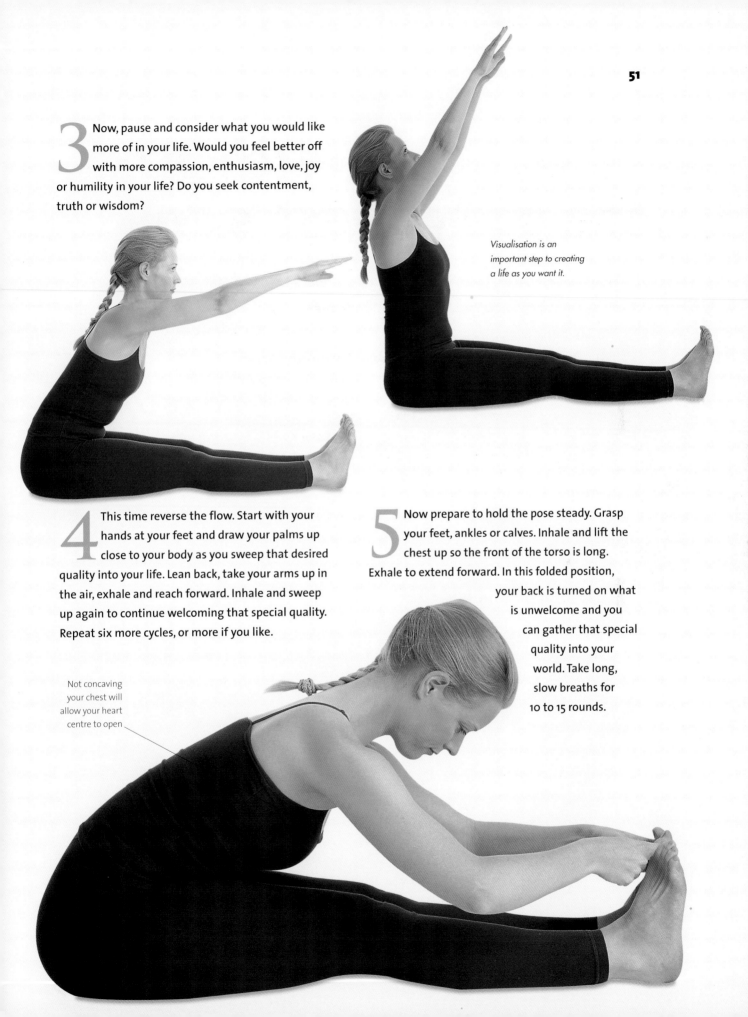

Purvottanasana Stretch on the body's east side

This is a counterpose for Paschimottanasana (see pages 50–51) and other forward bends.

1 Sit on the floor with your legs in front of you. Place the hands on the floor 15cm (6in) behind your hips, fingers pointing forwards. Point your toes away and lift your hips high. As you press your palms into the floor, fully expand your chest and release your neck and head back. Keep your front thigh muscles working and your toes pressing to the floor. Do three repetitions for five to ten breaths each.

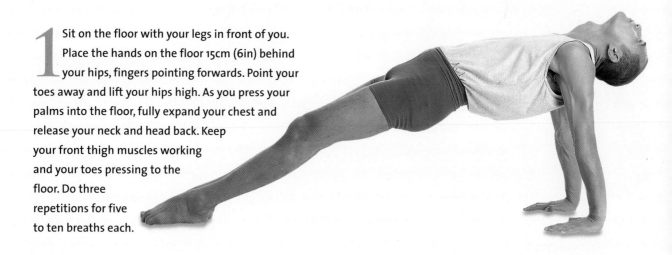

2 An easier variation is to begin with bent knees, then lift the hips and chest.

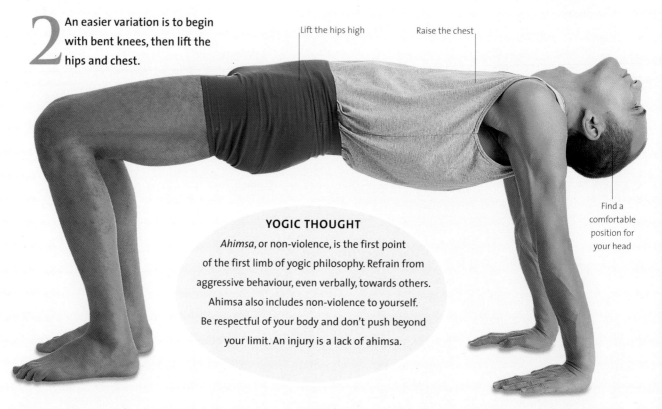

Lift the hips high

Raise the chest

Find a comfortable position for your head

YOGIC THOUGHT

Ahimsa, or non-violence, is the first point of the first limb of yogic philosophy. Refrain from aggressive behaviour, even verbally, towards others. Ahimsa also includes non-violence to yourself. Be respectful of your body and don't push beyond your limit. An injury is a lack of ahimsa.

Baddha konasana
Cobbler's pose

YOGIC THOUGHT

The quality of your posture is not measured by how flexible you are. Measure your pose by how steady your breath is.

Cobbler's pose promotes good health for the urinary and reproductive systems in men and women. It is especially helpful for women during pregnancy or for menstrual disorders.

1 Sit on the floor and bring the soles of your feet together with the heels near the perineum. Use the pressure of your hands to the floor behind you to tilt the pelvis forward, opening the inner thighs, groin and hips.

2 Although you want your knees as close to the floor as possible, don't force them down. They will release down more easily if you direct them out and back away from the root of the inner thigh.

3 If you can comfortably sit erect without the support of your hands behind you, hold your feet. If not, pressurise your hands on the floor, or sit on folded blankets. With your chest broad and open, breathe into the pose.

TIP
Don't bounce to release by butterflying your knees up and down. Learn to use the exhalation to soften the tight areas.

Let the elbows help ease the legs down

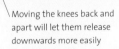

Moving the knees back and apart will let them release downwards more easily

4 If your pelvis tips forward easily, bend your elbows into the calves to ease the knees back and down closer to the floor and fold forward. Breathe evenly for five to ten rounds.

Upavista konasana sequence
Seated wide angle pose

As the connective tissue and muscle groups are large, it takes time for them to relax progressively into these forward stretches. In a single sitting, given time and patience you can stretch deeper than you imagined possible.

CAUTION
Ease off if you experience too much intensity on the inner thighs or pain in the inner knee.

1 Sit with your legs out to the sides at a 90 degree angle. Check that your kneecaps and toes are not rolling forwards or backwards, but point straight up to the sky. Twist to the right and take your left hand to your outer right knee. Cup your right hand on the floor behind you. This twist/pose prepares you for the wide-legged side stretch. Take five slow breaths. Feel your spine grow taller with each inhalation. On every exhalation feel your waist narrowing as you twist deeper.

TIP
In straight leg forward bends, keep your kneecaps and toes pointing directly up. You can even mark a dot at the centre of your knee to remind yourself!

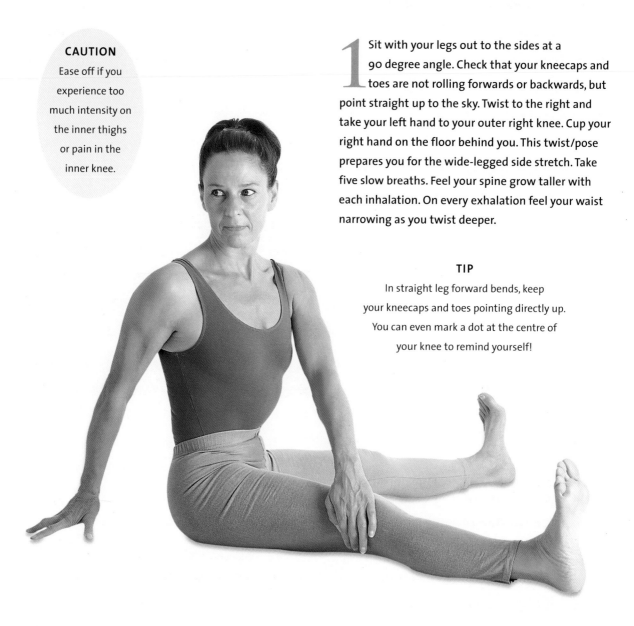

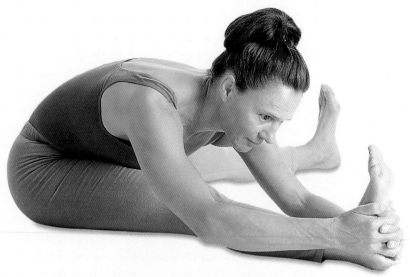

4 Inhale and create the sensation of the torso lifting out of the pelvis. Exhale and fold part way forward to grasp your calves, ankles or loop the big toes. Once more, inhale, lift up a little, lengthen from pubic bone to throat, then exhale out and down. Build to hold this for 20 breaths.

2 Untwist slightly so your breastbone is in line with your right thigh. Exhale and stretch forward to reach your right calf or foot. To work deeper into the pose, anchor your left seatbone down to the floor. Turn the toes back and extend through both heels. Hold this position for five to ten full breaths.

Bend your elbows as you ease yourself lower

3 Now you are ready for Upavista konasana. Sit up and press your fingertips to the floor behind you so your chest lifts and you tilt your pelvis forward. Just this movement alone will start to stretch the inner thigh and, if you have stiff hips, this may be as far as you go in this pose for today.

5 When you have completed both sides, support under your knees with your hands as you bring your legs together.

Gomukhasana
Cow-face pose

This pose is invaluable for relieving tight hips and shoulders. Poses we find most challenging are often the ones with the most to offer us.

1 Sit on the floor with your legs in front of you, knees bent up. Reach your right hand under your thigh to grasp your left ankle and pull it around to rest by your right hip. Now take your right foot over the top to rest by your left hip. In the complete pose, your right knee will stack up on top of the left.

2 Take your left arm straight up. Rotating from your shoulder, turn your little finger side to the front. Stretch up from your left hip to your fingertips, bend your elbow and lower your forearm behind you. Hold your elbow with your right hand and take several breaths as you ease your left hand further down your back. Now release your right arm down. Rotate from the shoulder so your thumb turns back. Bend the arm to grasp your hands together. Open your chest as you sit up tall for 10 to 15 breaths. Check that your head is straight, not tilting down or off to one side.

3 If you have tight shoulders, walk your hands together using a soft belt.

4 As an alternative, place your right ankle on your left knee. This helps to loosen tight hips.

TIP
If you find your top knee stays high in the air, use folded blankets to raise your seat.

This step 4 alternative offers an easier option

Navasana **Boat pose**

Strengthening the abdomen often helps back conditions, too. Develop your strength until you can hold Navasana for three rounds.

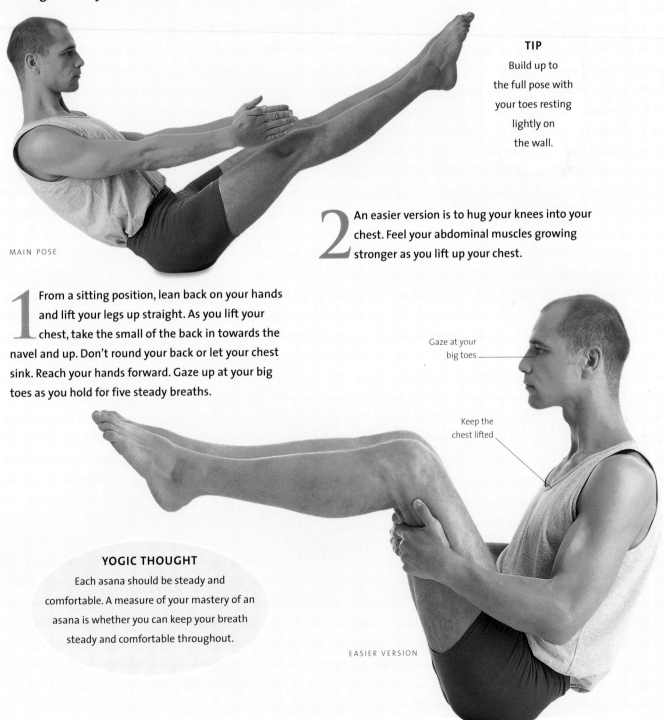

MAIN POSE

TIP
Build up to the full pose with your toes resting lightly on the wall.

2 An easier version is to hug your knees into your chest. Feel your abdominal muscles growing stronger as you lift up your chest.

1 From a sitting position, lean back on your hands and lift your legs up straight. As you lift your chest, take the small of the back in towards the navel and up. Don't round your back or let your chest sink. Reach your hands forward. Gaze up at your big toes as you hold for five steady breaths.

Gaze at your big toes

Keep the chest lifted

YOGIC THOUGHT
Each asana should be steady and comfortable. A measure of your mastery of an asana is whether you can keep your breath steady and comfortable throughout.

EASIER VERSION

Bhujapidasana
Arm pressure balance

You probably don't require more arm strength than you already have to do this balance. Instead, concentrate on your mental focus in order to balance yourself.

2 Lean forward, bend your elbows to 90 degrees, and walk your feet forward towards each other. Lift up through the abdominal region as raise your head to gaze forwards, and lift your feet up in the air to cross the ankles. Extend the arms and hold for five breaths. Rest down and repeat with your feet crossed the opposite way.

1 Stand with the feet hip width apart, and bend forward. Take your right arm between and back through your legs. Place the hand on the floor by the outside of your right foot. Bend your knee and take as much of your upper arm behind it as you can so the back of your thigh touches high up on your upper arm. Place the palm flat on the floor, fingers facing forward. To do the same on the left side, you will have to squat to flatten both palms on the floor.

TIP

To give a counterstretch to the wrists and forearms after Bhujapidasana or Adho Mukha Svanasana (see pages 46–47), kneel and take the backs of your hands to the floor in front. Your wrists point away from you and your fingers towards your knees. Lean back.

Work to straighten the arms

Change the crossing of the ankles with each repetition

Twists

Imagine squeezing soapy water out of a dish sponge, and then immersing it to soak up fresh water. Yoga twists have a similar action on the abdominal organs. Twisting the trunk gives a gentle squeeze to the organs, flushing out deoxygenated blood and allowing fresh blood to enter and nourish the tissues.

This twisting pressure has a good massaging effect on the organs, too. The kidneys, liver, spleen and the digestive system all benefit from yoga twisting. Backaches are often relieved by twists.

Apart from being uplifting physically, spiralling the torso skywards gives a mental lift. As upward spirals of energy, twists increase vitality and boost energy. Twisting limbers the vertebral column, which, apart from housing important nerves, nudges the subtle energies upwards to higher centres.

If you feel 'wound up' by the challenges of life, enjoy the feeling of unwinding as you come out of the twist. So much time is spent as a human 'doing' rather than a human 'being'. Now, in untwisting, you have an opportunity to undo. Let yourself 'be' as you unwind and melt away unnecessary layers which have become superimposed on your body.

Those with heavy or painful periods can focus more on forward bends and proceed very gently with the twists. Avoid twists in cases of diarrhoea and severe colitis.

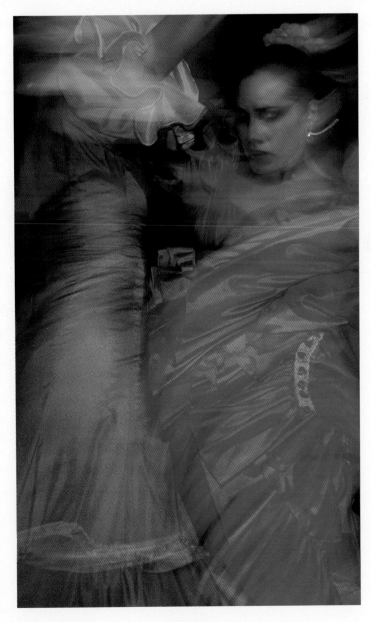

Spiralling upwards to the sky gives an energy boost

Sukhasana Twist
Cross-legged twist

While this pose seems simple, it can teach us a lot about twisting correctly.

1 Sit cross-legged, with your left hand on your right knee and your right hand cupping the floor behind you.

2 The correct twisting action begins at the root of your back. Learn to work in segments as you move the twist progressively up your spine.

3 Press your fingertips to the floor and inhale taller. To begin the twist, exhale and shunt your lower abdominal muscles to the right. On the next exhalation, move your middle abdominal muscles right. Visualise an upward spiral of energy. Each time you inhale, feel a lengthening upwards of your spine, and on each exhalation, twist deeper. Involve your upper abdominal muscles in the twist.

4 Remembering to use at least one breath per section, turn your ribs to the right, and involve your arms to help you twist. Then exhale the shoulders around. Keep your head facing the front as in this position your body feels safer to twist to your maximum. Finally, turn your head right to find the position which feels right for your neck. Hold for five to ten breaths, energy spinning upwards, before unwinding.

5 Take a moment to feel the effects that the twist has had on your abdomen, your ribs, the rest of your body and your mind. Twist to side two, then change the crossing of the legs and repeat both sides.

6 Don't bend the spine back and jam the floating ribs forward. Keep your back straight so your head and neck are over your pelvis. Both shoulders and both ears are the same height from the floor.

TIP

As your back releases tension and lengthens upwards, you might seem to twist less, but it will be a better quality twist than if your back were to stay short.

Marichyasana II **Sage twist**

As you breathe deeply in this pose, the pressure of your thigh against your abdomen will gently massage your abdominal organs.

TIP
As twists tend to compress one lung slightly, be aware of the other lung being exercised fully as it fills with air.

1 Sit with your legs in front of you. Bend your right knee up and bring your heel close to your buttock. To begin the twist, press into the floor with your right hand, lean back and reach your left hand up to the sky. Take a few breaths to lengthen the left side of the torso.

2 Now exhale, lean forwards and wedge your left elbow by your outer right knee. If possible, slide your left arm away so it contacts your right knee closer to your armpit. Use the instructions in the previous pose, cross-legged twist (see opposite), to twist upwards in stages. Hold five to ten breaths, then untwist, recentre, and repeat on the other side.

3 For the full posture, reach your left arm forwards beyond your right knee. Rotate from your shoulder to turn your arm thumb down and wrap it all the way around your knee to clasp your hands together. Grasp a soft belt if necessary.

Jathara parivartanasana Stomach strengthening twist

If you practise regularly, weak abdominal muscles will grow noticeably stronger in a short time.

1 Lie on your back with your arms out to the sides, hands at shoulder level. Bring both legs up in the air. Lift the hips and 'bunny hop' the buttocks to the left. Stretch out through your heels as you hold the left leg steady and exhale your right leg out to the side, toes aiming to fingertips. On your next exhalation, slowly lower your left leg to join the right. Inhale your left leg back to vertical. Inhale and follow with your right leg. Complete five repetitions on each side.

Stretch both heels away

2 For the full pose, exhale to lower both straight legs to the right. If you can, catch hold of your feet. Stretch both heels away, especially the top one, as you twist your abdominal muscles to the left. Anchor as much of the left side of your trunk to the floor as you can. Turn your head to gaze at your left hand. Hold for five breaths before inhaling both legs up. Do five repetitions on each side. Bend the knees to reduce the difficulty.

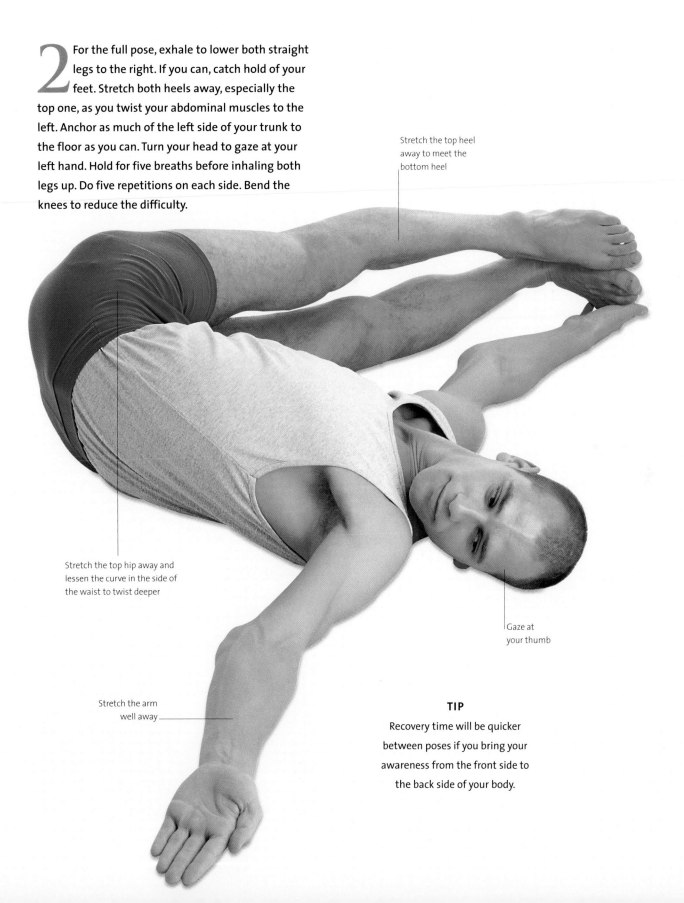

Stretch the top heel away to meet the bottom heel

Stretch the top hip away and lessen the curve in the side of the waist to twist deeper

Gaze at your thumb

Stretch the arm well away

TIP
Recovery time will be quicker between poses if you bring your awareness from the front side to the back side of your body.

Inversions

When you feel stuck, or in need of inspiration, it helps to see the world from another angle. Releasing the pressure of an everyday reality – gravity – can help lighten the mind too. An upside down position is an opportunity to consider things from a different point of view.

When you are inverted, blood flows more easily to the upper body. Endocrine glands like the pituitary and the hypothalamus in the brain, and the thyroid and parathyroid at the throat, get bathed in blood, so inverted poses play a role in balancing the hormones. Cerebral function is aided due to this extra nourishment, and inversions help combat tiredness and lethargy.

Inversions are a form of aerobic exercise too. Blood flows more easily to the heart, and consequently the heart fills more quickly and increases its activity to pump the blood back out. Good circulation is vital for true health. Improving the circulation can help many health conditions. Digestive function is stimulated, too, as the weight from above the intestines is lifted off.

Inversions have calming after effects, helping to quieten the body and mind. As they cool the system after the warming asana practice, they are generally performed at the end.

For some conditions, inversions may not be advisable. If you have high blood pressure, a neck problem, eye, ear or sinus problems, you should seek advice from a medical practitioner or experienced yoga teacher before beginning inversions. Inversions are not advisable during menstruation, as blood flow may be altered.

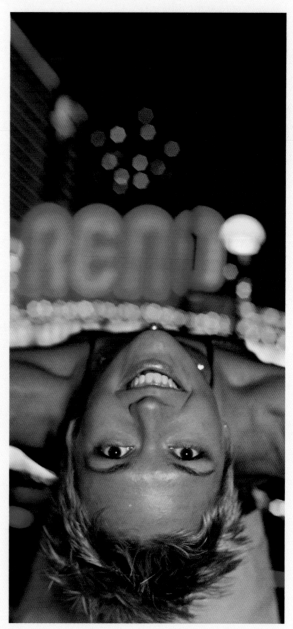

Blood flow to the upper body is increased when you are upside down.

Sarvangasana
Shoulderstand

The shoulderstand stimulates circulation to the thyroid and parathyroid glands, and regulates blood flow to the head. You can practise this pose for many minutes to experience its deeply calming effects (see caution on page 66).

1 Take three blankets and fold them three times. Lie on your back over the neatly lined up edges of the blankets. Your head will be on the floor, and your shoulders on the blankets, 5cm (2in) away from the edge.

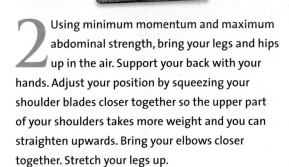

2 Using minimum momentum and maximum abdominal strength, bring your legs and hips up in the air. Support your back with your hands. Adjust your position by squeezing your shoulder blades closer together so the upper part of your shoulders takes more weight and you can straighten upwards. Bring your elbows closer together. Stretch your legs up.

3 Keep your neck straight; never turn it from side to side. Shoulderstand is not called neck stand, and for good reason! Although it might look as if the neck is taking a lot of weight, the neck muscles need to stay relatively soft. If possible, ask a friend to feel the muscles on either side of your neck to check they are not strained. Redness or strain in the face means it's time to come down and rest. Build your time in the pose from one to ten minutes.

4 To come down, hinge at the hips and lower your feet a little over your head. Release your hands, and lower your legs with control. Lying flat, turn your head to the left and right a few times to release your neck. Move off the blankets and hug your knees to your chest and rock slowly from side to side. Lie quietly and feel the effects of the pose on your body. Matsyasana (see page 39), a twisting pose and a forward bend feel nice after Sarvangasana.

Shoulderstand
against the wall

If you have trouble getting into
a shoulderstand, this safe and controlled
variation gives the same benefits.

TIP

Hold the skin on
your back rather
than your clothes
for a steadier
pose.

1 Put three tri-folded
blankets about
20–30cm (8–12in)
away from the wall. Sit in
front of them with your side
and one hip touching the
wall. Use your hands
for support and ease
yourself around to
lean back on your
elbows and bring
your legs up the
wall. Lift your head
to ensure your body is
straight. When you lie
down, your shoulders should be 5cm (2in)
away from the edge of the blankets and
your head on the floor.

3 To lift your hips up, press your feet into
the wall. Support your back with your
hands. Open your groin to move your
hips forward, lining up your hips and knees
over your shoulders.

4 If you wish to go further, straighten your
legs to bring your feet to the wall one by one.
If you feel comfortable, bring your legs away
from the wall one at a time.
To come down, reverse the steps.

2 Bend your knees so that
your feet are completely
flat to the wall.

CAUTION

Shoulder stand and Halasana should
be avoided in menstruation or in some ear or
eye problems, e.g. detached retina or glaucoma.
For heart problems, high blood pressure,
previous neck injuries or pregnancy,
seek professional advice.

Halasana **Plough pose**

This upside down forward bend soothes the nerves. It has the same effects and contraindications as Sarvangasana or shoulderstand (see pages 65–66).

1 From shoulder stand, lower your legs overhead. If your toes touch the floor, stretch your arms along the floor, and, if possible, interlace your fingers. Stretch your arms and legs in opposite directions. If your toes can't reach the floor, support your back with your hands. Build up to hold this pose for five minutes.

2 A more restful version is to roll back down slightly from the tops of your shoulders, widen and soften across your upper back, and lay your arms passively on the floor behind your head.

3 Slowly roll down to come out of Halasana. Use your abdominal muscles to lower both legs until your are lying flat. Rest for a while. Matsyasana (see page 39) is a complementary pose to do after Halasana.

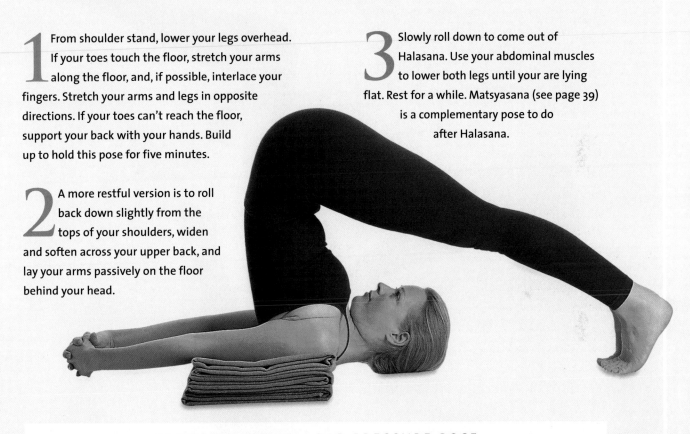

KARNAPIDASANA — EAR PRESSURE POSE

Stretch the spine as you cocoon yourself into this posture. From Halasana, bend your knees to your ears. If possible, have the tops of your feet to the floor, otherwise tuck your toes under. Hold your back with your hands. To deepen the pose, stretch both arms along the floor behind you and interlace your fingers. Alternatively, wrap your arms over the back of your knees. Hold this pose for five to ten breaths before coming back to Halasana.

From **Halasana** to **Paschimottanasana**

1 If you are on a flat cushioned surface, then enliven the spine by rolling between these poses. As you do, maintain a relaxed back and shoulders. Slow it down to enjoy the feeling of massaging the muscles all the way along the spine and shoulders.

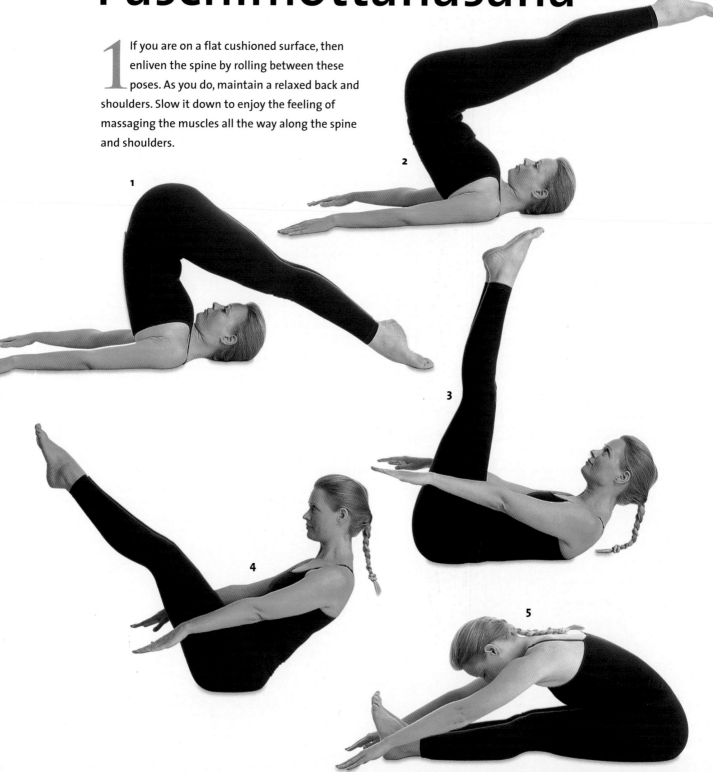

Relaxation

The role of deep relaxation in deep healing should never be underestimated. It is a generous act, not a selfish one, to give yourself restorative time. Relaxing fully lets you emerge refreshed and vibrant to participate in a wonderful, positive life. You will be better able to give more, live more, laugh more and love more.

Yoga postures alter the *prana*, the body's vital force, which is involved in healing and revitalising the mind and body. During yoga relaxation, the prana built up by your asana practice is consolidated, so it's not dispersed and lost. Each asana session concludes with deep relaxation. In some ways it is the most important part of the practice so it should never be skipped. This time gives the body the opportunity after its work-out, to do its 'work-in'.

From the outside, deep relaxation looks as easy as taking a nap. In fact, many people find it the most difficult pose of all. Unlike sleeping, yoga relaxation is a conscious process of learning to undo tension. Each part of the body is first brought to mind, relaxed and the awareness of it maintained. Discipline is required to keep the mind alert as the body progressively relaxes.

You will find relaxation easier after you have extended yourself to your limit. Make a fist with one hand and keep it clenched for 10 seconds. Relax that fist and compare the feelings in the two hands. Most likely you feel more sensations in the hand that was clenched. In yoga, find the edge in each posture, fully occupying both muscles and mind. This process creates space for a lingering awareness once the tension is released. It becomes easier to tune into an area and let it deeply relax. As you develop the ability

to stay mentally present throughout your asana practice, full relaxation will come more easily.

Deep relaxation teaches us how to let go. So often we cling on to objects, people or ways of thinking. Relaxation is a time to withdraw from these attachments. Observe your thoughts, should they wander, then guide them gently back to the sensations of the body and let go of stored tension.

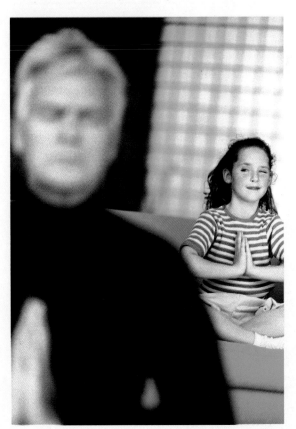

Complete relaxation will come eventually – it just takes practice.

Exploration Finding the right position for the yoga relaxation

It is important to be completely comfortable during the final relaxation. A few modifications may cater to any special needs your body may be experiencing during the practice.

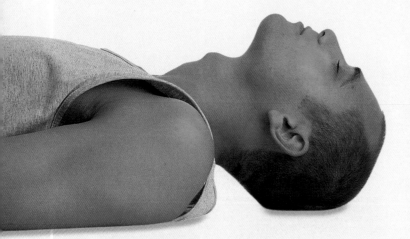

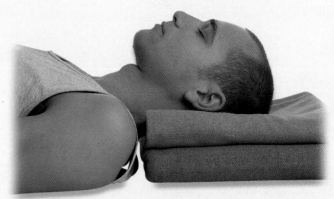

2 Use as many folded blankets as necessary to bring your chin and forehead level from the floor. When you have found the right position, your throat won't feel tense or constricted.

1 Find the best position for your head by having a friend observe you as you lie on your back. Ideally, your chin and forehead will be equal height from the floor. If your chin is higher than your forehead the back of your neck will tend to shorten.

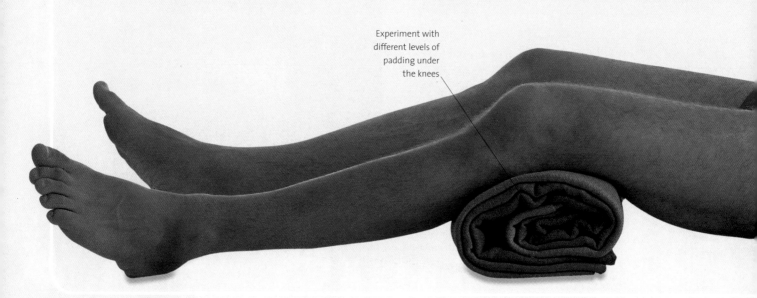

Experiment with different levels of padding under the knees

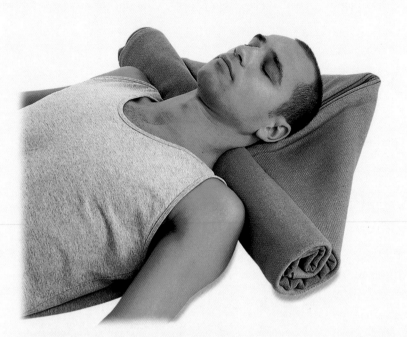

3 Make a neck pillow by folding a blanket three times. Roll up one side of the narrow edge to about half way. Fold in the two corners of the remaining flap to form a triangular shape for your head to rest on. The natural inward curve of the neck should feel completely supported against the firm roll. Lie down to test the height and adjust the size if necessary. Your chin and forehead should be level, and the same height from the floor. Depending on the natural curve in your neck, you might need to raise the level of your head, or lower it by unfolding the triangular flap.

4 When lying flat, the lower back will naturally curve away from the floor. However, If you have an exaggerated curve in the lower back, or a back problem, you might benefit by bending your knees. Place wide pillows or a bolster under your knees to allow the lower back to move a little closer towards the floor.

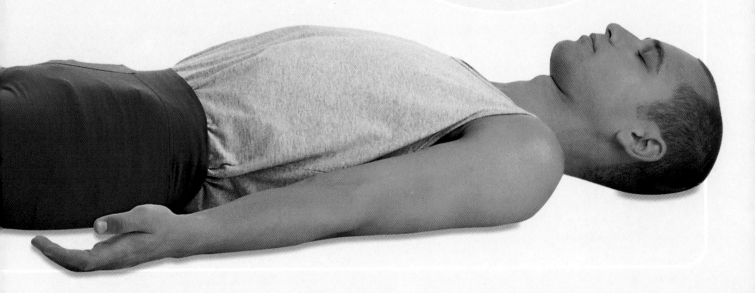

Savasana **Corpse pose**

While this pose looks like the easiest of all the yoga asanas, it is actually one of the hardest to master as the mind needs to stay present while the body lets go. Take at least five minutes in relaxation for every 30 minutes you have spent practising asanas. Ask a friend to read this technique aloud slowly.

1 Lie on your back with your legs a little apart and feet out to the sides. Take your hands a little away from the hips, palms facing upwards, fingers softly curling. Raise your head and look down your body to check the symmetry between left and right sides. Lower your head and close your eyes.

2 Allow five or ten minutes to soften each part of your body systematically. Sweep your mind over your body from toes and fingertips to the crown of your head. Don't skip anywhere; as you become aware of each part, and where there is tension, relax it.

3 Finally, bring your awareness to your face and scalp. Relax your mouth by slightly separating bottom lip from top. Take your tongue away from the roof of your mouth and let it float in the centre. Feel your jaw muscles release. As your eyes relax, your eyeballs will seem to sink deeper into their sockets. Release any holding in your eyelids, your forehead. Soften the skin on your face so it feels as though any lines smooth out and disappear.

YOGIC THOUGHT
Remember that yoga is not just doing postures, and your yoga practice doesn't have to end here. Integrate yoga into your life by going about your daily life with awareness and consciousness.

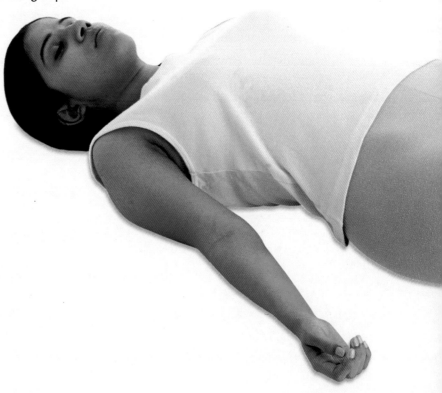

4 Now that each part of your body is relaxed, mentally commit yourself to staying perfectly still until your relaxation is complete. As with meditation (see page 86), any outer movement will distract you from your inner world. Keep your mind alert, observe the sensations in the body. Your body progressively lets go. Give permission for your emotional body to let go, too. Each exhalation brings a deeper relaxation, so the body feels heavier, as if sinking into warm earth. Each inhalation distributes life force to all the cells in the body. Should your mind wander, gently bring it back to the delicate breath. The more you focus mentally on this process, the deeper you will go.

DEEPEN IT

Exaggerating muscle tension raises your level of awareness. Work through the body, tensing each section of the body for a few seconds, to allow a deeper surrendering into the relaxation.

TIP

Use visualisation to fill your body with positive energy. Choose a colour which connotes a healing energy. With each breath, inhale this coloured light into your centre. Each inhalation will brighten this light, while each exhalation increases its density at your core, until it begins to expand outwards to fill the rest of your body. Pay particular attention to filling up any weaker area with this positive energy. Inhale your whole body so full with the light that it spills over the edges and floats around you. Know that when you come out of the relaxation, you will always have your breath as a tool, any time you need it.

5 When it's time to come out of Savasana, deepen your breath. Each inhalation fills your body with energy until your eyes, energised from inside, naturally want to blink open. Take one arm overhead and roll over to curl up on that side. When you are ready, slowly come up to sit quietly.

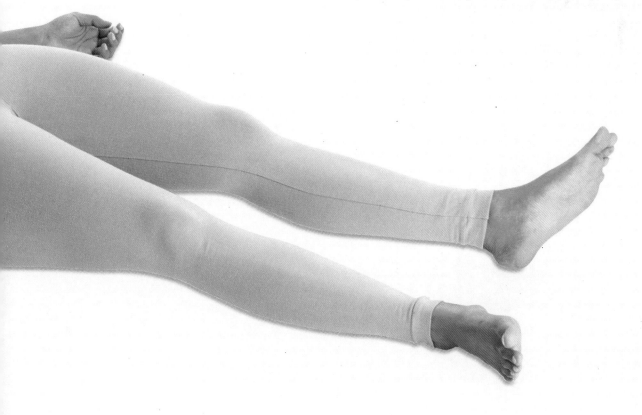

Relaxation breaks

Use these poses to relax and renew whenever you wish during your practice, or throughout your day. Sprinkling your asana practice with these poses gives a quiet receptive space to receive feedback from your body.

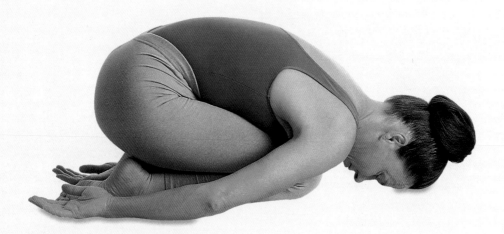

BALASANA **CHILD POSE**
Sit on your heels with your knees together. Fold forward to lay your torso on your thighs. Bring your forehead to the floor and rest the backs of your arms on the floor. Soften your shoulders, close your eyes and follow your breath.

A variation is to keep your big toes together as you spread your knees apart and stretch your arms forward along the floor. If you have high blood pressure, or if your buttocks don't release down close to your heels, modify the pose. Stack two fists up and rest your forehead on them.

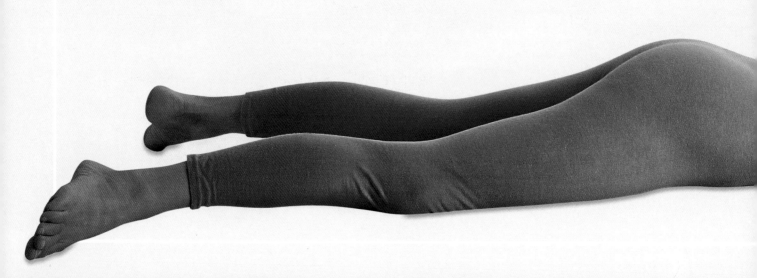

VIPARITA KARANI **RESTORATIVE INVERSION**

Viparita Karani literally means against the grain, as the normal flow of the circulation in the legs is altered. Do it daily for 15 minutes if you have varicous veins. You can restore in this pose without the blankets too.

Fold two or three blankets four times and place them 8cm (3in) out from the wall. Sit on them, side on, with one hip to the wall. Support yourself with your hands, as you swivel around to lay yourself down. Straighten your legs up the wall. Have your buttocks as close to the wall as possible. Lift your head up to make sure your trunk is perpendicular to the wall. Have your arms a little out from your sides, palms facing up. Lie quietly, eyes closed, observing the rhythm of your breath.

TIP
Uttanasana (see pages 28–29) and Adho Mukha Svanasana (see pages 46–47) are useful poses for recentring.

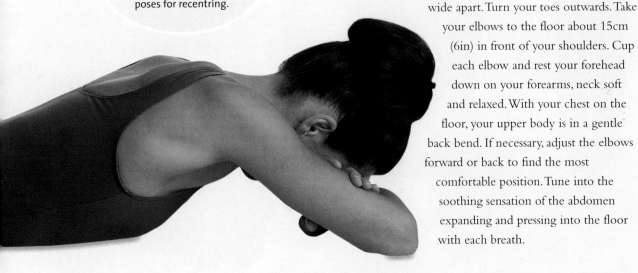

MAKRASANA **CROCODILE POSE**

Gentle pressure on the forehead relaxes the frontal lobe of the brain which helps quieten and soothe.

Lie on your front with your feet comfortably wide apart. Turn your toes outwards. Take your elbows to the floor about 15cm (6in) in front of your shoulders. Cup each elbow and rest your forehead down on your forearms, neck soft and relaxed. With your chest on the floor, your upper body is in a gentle back bend. If necessary, adjust the elbows forward or back to find the most comfortable position. Tune into the soothing sensation of the abdomen expanding and pressing into the floor with each breath.

Surya Namaskar
Sun Salutation

The flowing folding and unfolding of sun salutation is a great warm-up. A single breath carries you into each pose. Start with three rounds and build to six, offering each one up like a prayer.

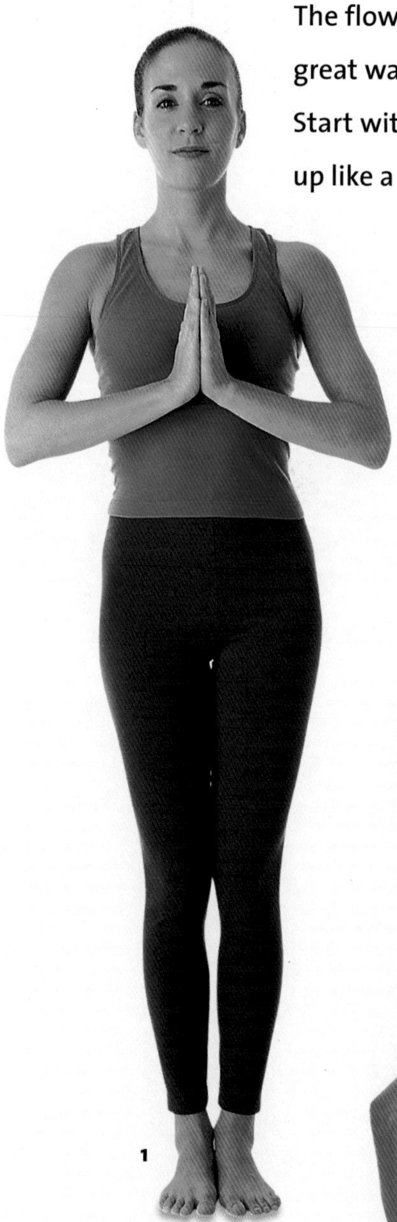

1 Stand in Samasthiti pose (see page 22), hands in prayer.

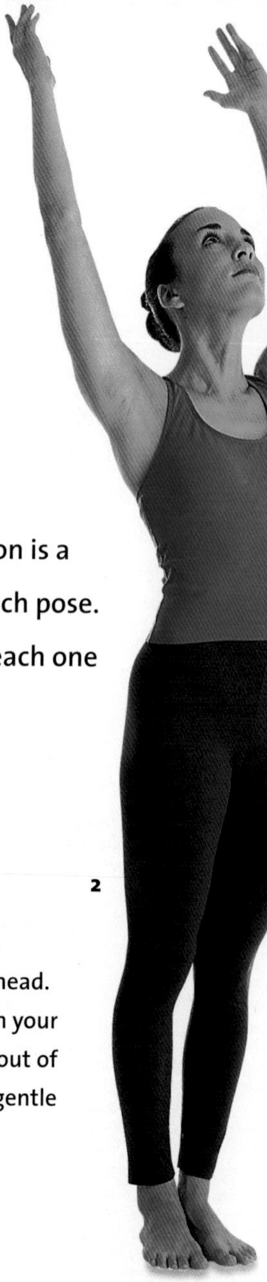

2 Inhale and take your arms overhead. Ground through your feet, lift up your torso out of your hips and make a gentle back bend.

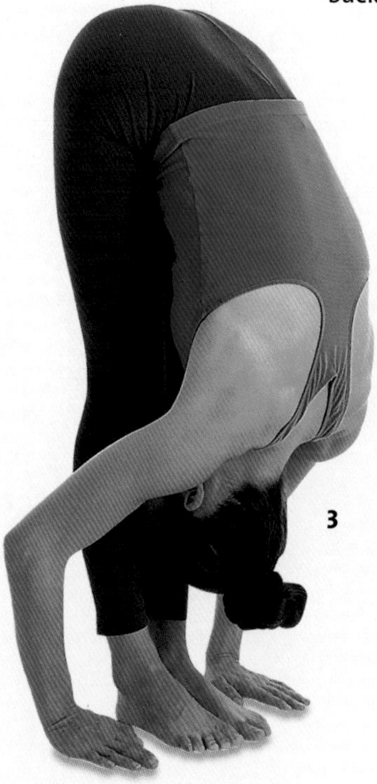

3 Exhale and fold forwards to Uttanasana (see pages 28–29). Bend your knees, if necessary, to bring your finger tips or even palms to the floor.

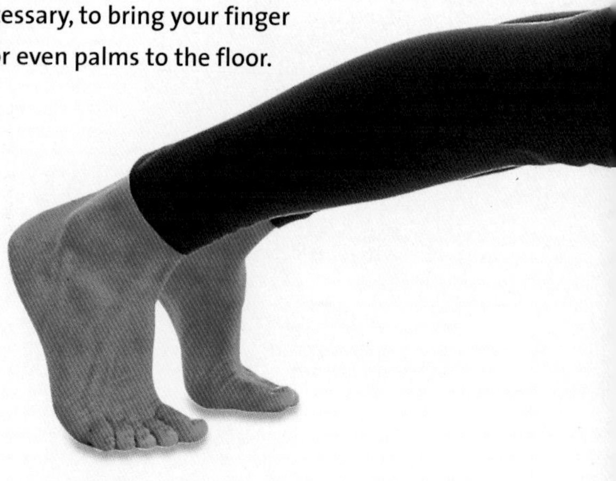

1

2

3

4 Inhale and look forward as you step your right leg back to lunge, knee to the floor. Press your fingertips to the floor as you lift your chest away from your left thigh.

TIP
Vary your sun salutation by holding each pose for three breaths. This gives you time to feel your way into the pose and deepen it.

5 Exhale and step your left leg back so your body makes a straight line from heels to head.

6 Inhale as you bring your knees to the floor. Then exhale as you lower your chest and chin to touch the floor.

7 Inhale as you roll up to the cobra (see page 36).

8 Exhale to downward-facing dog (see pages 46–47).

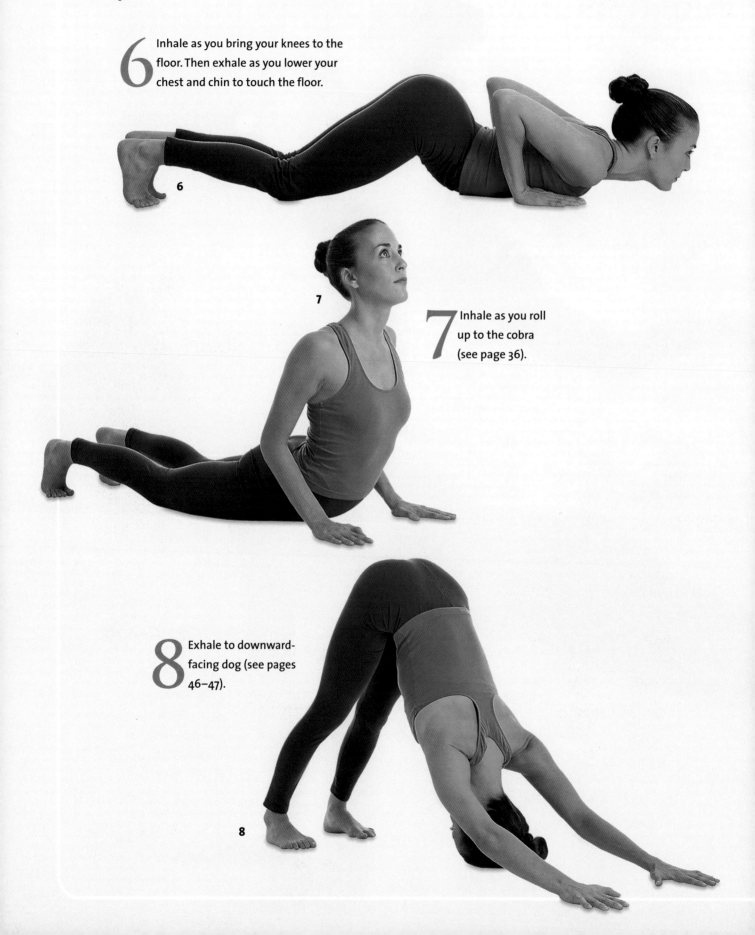

9 Inhale and step your right leg forward.

10 Exhale, step your left leg forward and fold into Uttanasana.

11 Inhale and firm your front thigh and abdominal muscles as you stand to reach your arms overhead.

12 Exhale to Samasthithi. Inhale and repeat on the left side.

Pranayama Yoga breathing

When we feel very alive, we really mean we have lots of energy. One fount of energy is the food we eat. Another is the ideas we have. A third source is the breath.

Breath, life and energy are all interconnected. Yogis have a single word for all three – *prana*. This vital force is what is transmitted during 'hands on' healing such as reiki. It is the aura that can be recorded using Kirlian photography. The energy points along the spine known as chakras are storehouses for prana. When prana leaves the body, death occurs. When pranic levels are high, the body will be completely charged with energy.

Pranayama may be translated as 'pranic capacity' or as 'control of the prana'. It uses the breath to affect the physical, mental, emotional and spiritual bodies.

Breathing lies under the control of the medulla oblongata, the 'primitive' brain stem. This breath is regarded as involuntary; it happens automatically. In conscious breathing, a more evolved part of the brain, the cerebral cortex, is activated. Pranayama, in making an involuntary process more voluntary, has profound physiological, psychological and spiritual effects.

Deep, conscious breathing and full expansion of the lungs is a powerful energising tool. As more oxygen is distributed to the tissues, all cellular processes are enhanced to better repair, digest, detoxify and combat disease. Optimally nourished cells make up a fully healthy body.

The breath is connected with the mind. A shock makes you hold your breath. If you feel excited, your breath is fast, shallow and irregular. When your mind is at ease, the breath becomes slow, deep and rhythmic. Calming the breath will quiet the mind.

Conscious breathing is a bridge between the nervous system, mind and emotions. Pranayama boosts mental energy and increases mental clarity. It deepens awareness, assists coping and decreases emotional fluctuations.

Spiritually, pranayama expands consciousness. It increases self-awareness towards the ultimate goal of yoga – self-realisation. Sensory cravings and distractions are reduced. The normally outward looking senses are drawn inwards.

Pranayama needs to be practised daily for the effects to be seen. If your practice includes asanas, do these first, then Savasana. Then practise pranayama and finally refresh in Savasana for 10 minutes.

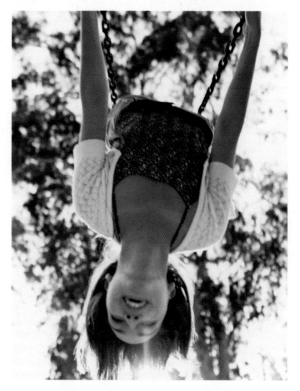

Deep conscious breathing reinvigorates body and soul.

Exploration Finding a

comfortable position for Pranayama

Some believe certain positions for pranayama and meditation are 'better' than others. But really, the best position is the one that is the steadiest and most comfortable for you, as long as it keeps the back, neck and head in a straight line. Any strain felt in the body will flow over to affect the breath adversely, so being comfortable is important.

The beauty of pranayama is that absolutely everyone can do it. The only requirement for practice is being able to breathe. If you are physically weak or ill, you can do pranayama lying down. Better still, bend your knees up and lean them in together. Take your feet wider than your hips, toes turned in. This position is supremely comfortable and you are less likely to fall asleep. If you feel yourself dozing off, separate the knees.

A classical posture, Padmasana – Lotus Pose – where the legs are crossed and both feet sit soles up on the thighs, is advisable only if you have extremely flexible hips. When the hips are tight, the knees risk injury. Most westerners, who grow up sitting on chairs rather than sitting cross-legged on the floor, require dedicated hip opening work before they can sit comfortably in Padmasana. This posture is not used in this book.

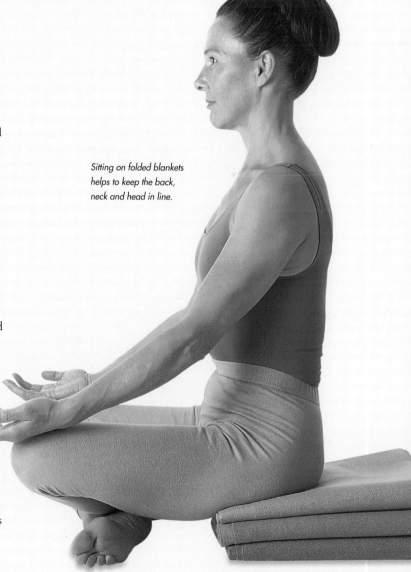

Sitting on folded blankets helps to keep the back, neck and head in line.

SUKHASANA **COMFORTABLE POSE**

Cross your ankles, then slide your feet apart so that each foot comes to rest underneath the opposite knee. To sit at length and remain comfortable in this position, your knees must be level with or lower than your hips. If your knees are much higher than your hips, or if you find your upper body tilting backwards, sit on as many cushions as you need.

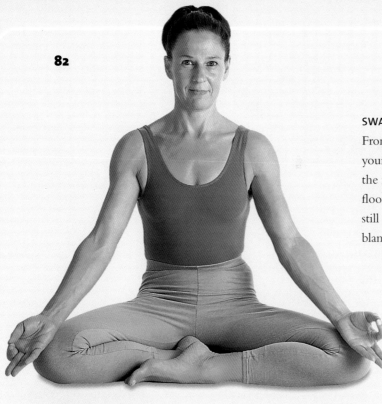

SWASTIKASANA FOLDED LEG POSE

From sitting, fold one leg in so your heel touches your perineum. Line up your other heel in front of the first one. Your knees will rest down towards the floor more easily than with Sukhasana, but you may still be more comfortable using a cushion or folded blanket to raise your seat.

SITTING ON A CHAIR

Choose a chair that you won't sink down into. Sit erect with your shoulders in line over your hips, not leaning into the backrest. Shorter people can rest their feet on a support, such as a rolled blanket. Experiment with a blanket folded several times to make a long pad and laid across the knees. When you place your hands palms up on the blanket, your elbows will be more at right angles and the extra height brings softness to the palms. This roll can be used in any of the seated poses.

VAJARASANA FIRM POSE

Kneel with your knees and ankles together and sit down on your heels. As you bring your weight down, your inner ankles will tend to splay apart. Keep them as close together as possible. If you are on a hard surface, you may like to pad under the tops of your feet with a soft support.

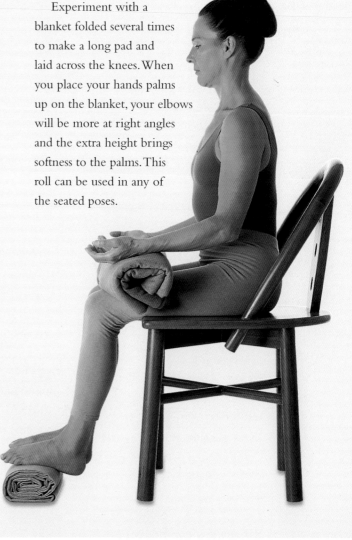

Ujjayi Pranayama

The Ujjayi breath gives control over the flow of air into the lungs
so that the breath becomes steadier, deeper and longer.
More oxygen is made available, enhancing the purification
and nourishment of each and every cell.

*Ujjayi breathing will focus
your mind and enhance
your asana practice.*

Ujjayi breathing is a little like drinking air through a straw. The glottis in the pharynx at the back of the mouth is partially closed. Friction is produced when air moves through the larynx, increasing the heat in body. This allows the body to stretch very deep into the asanas, so Ujjayi is an ideal way to breathe during your yoga practice. Practice Ujjayi for 10 to 20 breaths while sitting. Take breaks when you need and finish with Savasana (see page 72). As your comfort with Ujjayi grows, expand it for the duration of your asana practice.

• Sit comfortably and take several exhalations, each time making a long 'haaaa' sound through your mouth.

• Close your mouth midway through the exhalation, but continue to make the 'haaaa' with your lips together. It will become a soft throaty sound that you can feel at the larynx. To check if you've got it, cover your ears with your palms and listen to the internal sound. It will have an ocean-like quality.

• Now open your mouth again and make this 'haaaa' while breathing in. Close your mouth midway through again, to leave a soft friction in your throat. Once again, the sound will be like the ocean.

TIP
You should feel no stress as you breathe. Trying 'too hard' changes the lungs, diaphragm, and nervous system which in turn will adversely affect the rest of your body and mind. Evenness in the breath will lead to evenness of temperament. Mentally follow your exhalation its entire length. Don't allow your boredom to let you lose awareness of it. Don't let your impatience make you rush on to a new breath before the present one is fully exhaled.

• Continue the internal 'haaaa' as you inhale and exhale through your nose. It's not necessary to breathe loudly or aggressively. This breath is soft in nature and volume. While the sound produced will be audible to someone close by, it's not necessary to fill the whole room. The quality of the Ujjayi breathing is not measured in volume, but in length and steadiness. Rather, bring your awareness to the constancy that this breath gives you. Each inhalation extends in a long, fluid way to deeply fill the lungs. Likewise the flow of air through your nostrils is slow and steady for the entire duration of the out-breath.

Nadi Shodhana Pranayama
Alternate nostril breathing

Working on the physical, mental and spiritual levels, this is a valuable pranayama. It acts as a purification (*shodhana*) of the subtle energy meridians (*nadis*) and balances two important pranic pathways. As it helps balance the nervous system and calm the mind, it is useful when you feel uptight or confused.

• Sit comfortably with your eyes closed. Curl the index and middle fingers of your right hand into your palm.
• Inhale fully through your nose. Close your right nostril with the thumb of your right hand and exhale fully through your left nostril.
• Inhale through the left side. Close your left nostril with your third and little fingers, release your thumb and exhale through your right nostril, so that the air flows at a constant rate.
• Inhale through the right side. Close your right nostril and open your left nostril to exhale.

TIP
To help keep your breath steady, imagine there is a saucer of fine ash under your nose. If you inhale too greedily it will be sucked inside you. If you exhale too forcefully, it will end up all over your clothes.

TIP
Practise alternate nostril breathing before bedtime to help you get off to sleep.

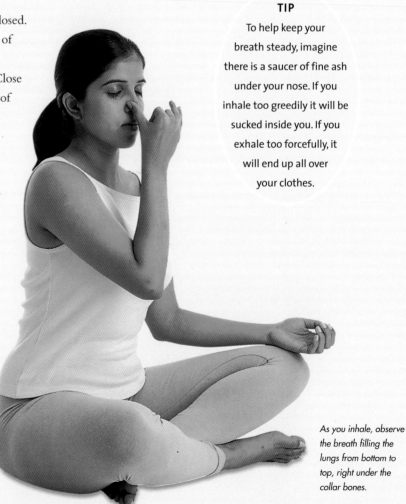

As you inhale, observe the breath filling the lungs from bottom to top, right under the collar bones.

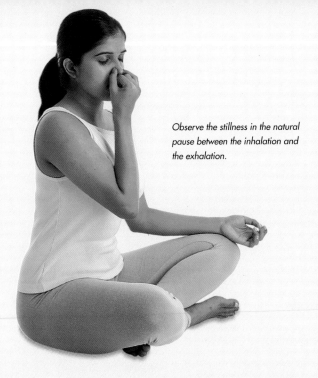

Observe the stillness in the natural pause between the inhalation and the exhalation.

Each round contains three inhalations on each side, beginning and ending with an exhalation to the left side. To keep track, you can count with your thumb to your fingers on your left hand. Complete five rounds, resting your arm down, and taking as long as you need in between. Finish by relaxing in Savasana (see page 46).

During the practice, keep your right elbow raised to avoid tilting your head to one side or placing pressure on your chest which impedes the filling of the lungs. Usually one nostril feels more open than the other. Nostril predominance shifts at regular intervals throughout the day.

• Then inhale with your left nostril to exhale through the right. Each inhalation and exhalation keeps the flow of air through the nostrils at the same rate from beginning to end.
• Inhale right, then exhale left. The rate of flow at the end of the exhalation should be the same as that at the beginning of the exhalation.
• Inhale left, then exhale right.
• Inhale right and finish with a final exhalation through the left nostril.
• Lower your hand down and take as many easy breaths as you need. Observe the quiet stillness.
When you feel ready, begin the next round.

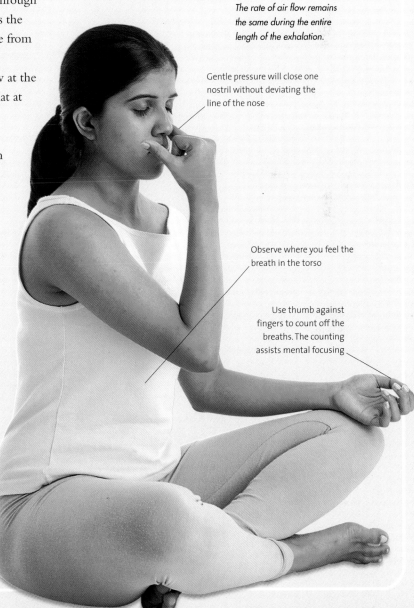

The rate of air flow remains the same during the entire length of the exhalation.

Gentle pressure will close one nostril without deviating the line of the nose

Observe where you feel the breath in the torso

Use thumb against fingers to count off the breaths. The counting assists mental focusing

DEEPEN IT

When you have practised this several times, implement a count. Inhale and exhale for a slow count of six beats each. When you become comfortable with this, increase it to eight. It should always feel natural, never tense. Force is counterproductive in pranayama so if you find yourself straining, then reduce the count. Using a count makes the length of the inhalation and exhalation equal and gives a mental point of focus that can quieten the constant chatter of the mind.

Meditation

On a cloudy day the sun seems a dull light behind a haze of white. When the sun can't be seen clearly, it's easy to forget, or doubt, its presence. Yet, the sun never stops shining. Meditation wipes away the cloudy veil – the false perceptions, the illusions – and makes you receptive to the touch of pure sunlight, the ever present bliss state.

During meditation the mind is alert and aware in a slow, effortless way. It is fixed solely on one point, to contemplate and become absorbed in the formless Self. As the Self integrates into the universal spirit, meditation is expansive. It is listening instead of doing, acting or imposing. It is observing and letting the mind be receptive to reality. Like wiping clean a dusty mirror, meditation opens you to perceive the true reflection of universal reality.

In the *Yoga-sutras*, an early text, yoga is defined as the restraint of the *chitta-vrtti* – the fluctuations of the mind. In the state of yoga modifications in the thought patterns will cease. Meditation helps to still the *chitta-vrtti*, and attain the state of yoga.

In a meditative state, the brain wave patterns change from the beta waves of the normal awake state, to the alpha waves of deeper relaxation. Regular meditators also show theta brain waves, which occur in a state of rest deeper than sleep, but in these states, the meditator is fully aware and conscious. As the two hemispheres of the brain synchronise, mental efficiency, cognitive and perceptual ability is increased –

Meditation can promote a deep sense of inner joy.

a study has even demonstrated meditation over a period of several years to increase the IQ.

Studies have shown impressive physiological effects of meditation. It has been shown to slow the aging process, lower blood pressure, decrease heart disease, breast cancer, osteoporosis and reduce stress related disorders such as insomnia and depression.

Stilling the mind is not an easy task. The Vedas, the earliest known compilations of Indian spiritual writings, say the mind is harder to control than the wind. Yet long-term meditators certainly feel that meditation improves their quality of life. It brings a sense of relief and recentring, like coming home after a long and difficult journey. Self-awareness deepens and perspective is gained. In some ways, day-to-day worries are transcended. There is an inner joy that comes with this superconscious state of detaching from worldly things and developing an objective observation. As during meditation you are aligning yourself with a positive, universal energy, something greater than yourself, meditation is a source of great inner strength.

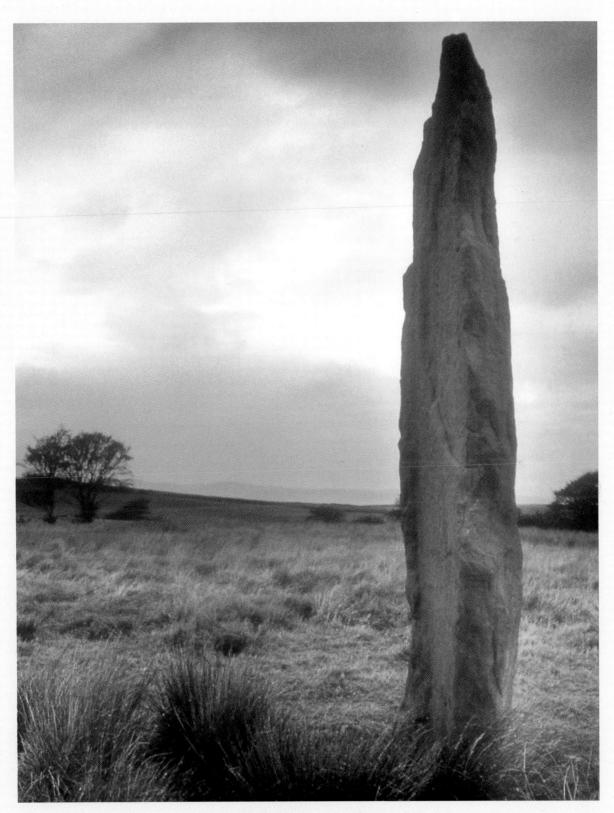

*Rather than doing or acting, meditation
allows us to simply observe what is.*

Five steps for **meditation**

Dedicate 20 minutes a day to your meditation practice, and you will reap the physiological, mental and emotional rewards.

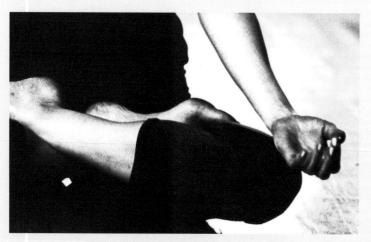

Sitting in the lotus position is for some the most comfortable way to meditate.

RELAX YOUR BODY

Yoga asana practice was originally designed to let the body sit comfortably in meditation. Short of a full asana practice, do a few stretches to increase your body awareness. Take a comfortable seated position with back, neck and head erect. (See the pranayama section, page 81, for instructions on how to sit.) If it feels right for you, offer a personal prayer, or chant to begin the session. Sweep your mind over your body, systematically relaxing each part from bottom to top. You can even do a full Savasana (see page 72) before sitting up to begin your meditation.

Once you have chosen your comfortable position, avoid further movement which will only act as a distraction. When you are sitting perfectly still, every physical sensation can feel like it is magnified. A small itch can become a huge torment. Breathe through these transitory sensations as they arise.

RELAX YOUR MIND

Take three cleansing breaths by inhaling through the nose and exhaling through the mouth. Use a sigh as you exhale to release fatigue or tension. Now practise three rounds of Nadi Shodhana pranayama (see page 84). Pay particular attention to the counting process. As with pranayama, strain is counterproductive to meditation. Keep the process relaxed.

INTERIORISATION

The breath or a mantra are useful tools to increase your concentration. You could use the ancient sound 'Om' to help focus your mind. Begin by chanting this mantra aloud, change to whispering it, then finally repeat it only in your mind.

If instead you choose to use the breath as your aid, begin by observing the flow of air through the nostrils. The cool air flows in though the nose, and the warmer air flows out. In time, follow the cool inhaled air from the nose, to the trachea. Continue to observe without any hurry. Don't alter your breath, simply be aware of what is. Possibly you can follow the flow as far down as your bronchial tubes and the lungs. On each exhalation, observe the warmed air flowing out through the nostrils from inside the body.

EXPAND YOUR CONSCIOUSNESS

The mind has random thoughts, spreading over many subjects. The concentration in stage three confined the thoughts to a single subject – a mantra or the breath. This next step further refines it. From having many thoughts on a single subject, there is now a single thought. Choose a subject on which you would like to expand your awareness, such as love or peace. The aim is not to prevent all thought, but to provide a focus point for the thoughts to revolve around. This one-pointed awareness is where meditation begins. Observe the flow of thought, like ripples in a lake, without following them. If you follow a thought that's not the focus of your meditation, you are lending it the energy to distract yourself. Practise mastery over the mind and gently bring your mind back to your chosen subject. The constant churning of the mindstuff gives way to peacefulness. In meditation you practise being the observer, not the doer.

CLOSING YOUR MEDITATION

Guide your thoughts to a higher aim such as the realisation of your true spiritual self. You might like to repeat a prayer or use a chant like the one at the start of this book (see page 6). Spiritual endeavours are of little use when not carried over into your day-to-day life. Let your calm and peaceful feelings spill into your encounters with others.

The benefits of meditation will spill over to your day-to-day life.

TIPS FOR MEDITATORS

• Set aside a regular time to meditate. Traditionally the best times of day to meditate are sunrise, noon, sunset or midnight.

• If you feel daunted by the whole process, then commit to sitting quietly for half an hour. During this time, just observe each thought, whatever comes, and let it go. Possibly, after about 15 minutes, your mind will come to you, begging for something to think about. This is when you can give it your chosen meditation topic to contemplate.

• If you have a busy mind, 'doing nothing' and just observing in meditation might make you feel bored. If so, accept it and make boredom the subject of that meditation.

• Any action, performed with mindfulness, can be meditative. A walking meditation is useful if you find sitting for long periods is very uncomfortable, or if you tend to fall asleep. Keep your eyes unfocused, gazing down to the floor. Walk slowly in a circle with your awareness on the feet. Feel the sensations in each sole as it rolls down to contact the floor, bears weight and then peels off the floor to take the next step. After this walking meditation, sit and continue the meditation.

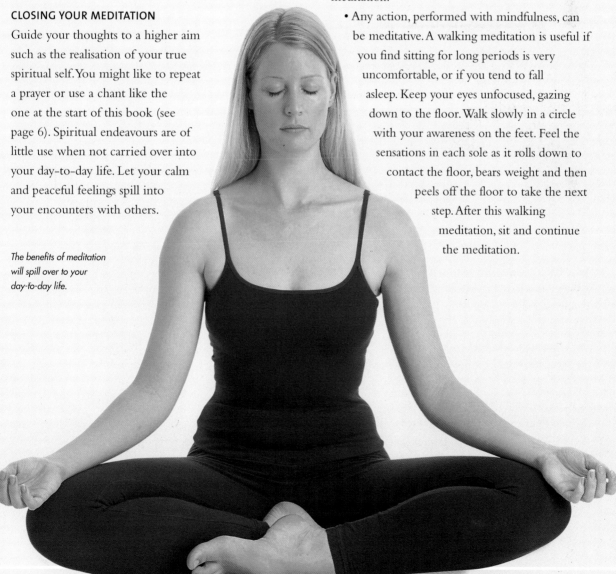

Therapeutic **yoga**

Real health lies beyond the standard medical definition of 'the absence of disease'. True health encompasses a state of supreme well-being and vitality on the physical, mental and spiritual levels.

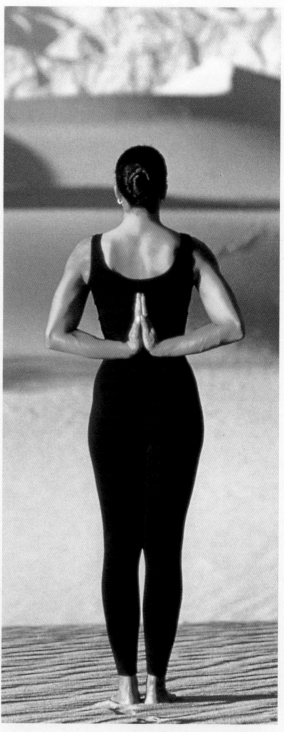

Regular pranayama and meditation help maintain mental and physical health.

Yoga assists in the cure of diseases in a variety of ways. Each asana has specific structural and functional effects on the body. Yoga asanas promote the natural pulsations in the body. These rhythms assist circulation, increasing vitality of each cell, tissue, organ and system.

Yoga helps to balance the hormonal and nervous systems. It balances the parasympathetic nervous system, involved in the 'restore and repair' response to aid healing.

Learning deep relaxation is curative on many levels. Regular pranayama and meditation assist the mental and emotional response of the person to their disease.

Yoga as therapy for disease takes a holistic approach, considering each person as an individual. Indians consider each person has five koshas, or sheaths: physical, pranic, mental, intellectual and bliss. Ill-health results from a disharmony in the koshas which yoga helps to rebalance. Each of the following common practices – cleansing techniques, postures, breath work, meditation, analysis, experience, chanting, devotion and relaxation – promotes health through its actions on one or more of the koshas.

This table on pages 92–93 shows suggested asanas for common ailments. A holistic approach aims to correct the cause of a condition and this information is intended as a guide only, not as a substitute for advice from a qualified medical practitioner.

COMMON AILMENTS AND CONDITIONS

If you suffer from one or more of the following common ailments or conditions, it is important to consider the following advice or consult a qualified health practitioner before practising yoga.

ARTHRITIS If it is difficult to hold a pose, don't stay long in it. Develop mobility in the joints by moving in and out of the pose with easy flowing movements. Avoid moving into the pain; use props if necessary.

ASTHMA Pranayama practice will retrain the breath. Back bends are useful as they lift and open the chest, encouraging fuller breathing. Avoid caving in the chest while practising forward bends.

ANXIETY Practise conscious breathing throughout the day to shift your thoughts from concerns and bring you back to the present. Physically work stress out with the asanas and perform them with as much mental focus as possible. After asanas, have a long savasana and perform Nadi Shodhana Pranayama.

CONSTIPATION Find the cause. Check your intake of fluid and dietary fibre are adequate. Sun salutation, inversions and twists stimulate the digestive system and encourage elimination.

DEPRESSION To help stay in the present moment, keep the eyes open during asana practice. Avoid forward bends as they tend to make you more introspective.

DIABETES Twists and back bends tone the pancreas. Yoga asanas increase circulation and overall vitality.

FATIGUE Rest mental fatigue with forward bends and savasana. Re-energise with pranayama.

HERNIATED SPINAL DISC Yoga can effectively manage slipped discs. Forward bending can seriously aggravate a slipped disc so hamstring flexibility needs to be developed and the back kept concave while bending forward. Support the area by strengtheniing the abdominal muscles.

HYPERTENSION Practise savasana, pranayama and meditation. Practise inversions and back bends only under the guidance of an experienced yoga teacher.

INSOMNIA Both mind and body rest more easily after being extended. Do energising asanas like Surya Namaskar and back bends in the mornings. If your practice is closer to bedtime, focus on forward bends and inversions. Take a long savasana.

IMMUNE SUPPORT After asana practice, take extra time for savasana and pranayama. While asana practice encourages health on the cellular level, savasana greatly assists healing on a deep level.

LOWER BACK STRAIN Lower back pain has many causes and it is essential to get a correct diagnosis. While bending backward may alleviate one condition, it could aggravate another. Work with an experienced teacher to find what is appropriate.

MENSTRUAL DISORDERS Back bends, forward bends, twists and Surya Namaskar increase vitality to the pelvis. Inverted postures help balance hormones.

YOGA DURING MENSTRUATION Inversions, strong twists and strong back bends should not be practised during menstruation. Forward bends and relaxation are recommended during this time.

YOGA FOR THE ELDERLY Although the poses might not be as extended as those shown here, performing them with awareness will bring the same benefits. Flowing into and out of poses, rather than holding them, will develop strength. Use props if necessary, eg. hold the wall for balance in standing postures.

OBESITY Sun salutation will help burn energy. Practise plenty of standing poses, back bends and inversions.

PREGNANCY Yoga can assist pregnancy and labour. If you are new to yoga, do not begin yoga in the first trimester. Attend a special pre-natal yoga class to learn the necessary asana modifications through the preganacy.

STRESS Some mental stress can be physically worked out in the asanas. Concentrating on body awareness during asana practice gives a mental break from worrying about other things. Long savasana releases mental and physical tension. Pranayama calms the nervous system.

THERAPEUTIC YOGA

This chart shows which asanas are helpful
for which conditions or ailments.

✿ Recommended

▲ Not recommended

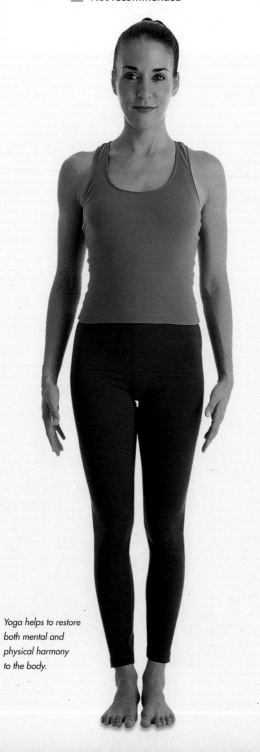

Yoga helps to restore both mental and physical harmony to the body.

	Cat pose	Awareness of breath	Standing poses	Bhujangasana
Arthritis	✿	✿	✿	✿
Asthma	✿	✿		✿
Anxiety	✿	✿		✿
Constipation		✿		
Depression			✿	✿
Diabetes		✿		
Fatigue				
Herniated spinal disc		✿		✿
Hypertension	✿	✿		▲
Insomnia				
Immune support				✿
Lower back strain	✿	✿	✿	
Menstrual disorders	✿			
Yoga during menstruation	✿	✿		
Yoga for the elderly	✿	✿	✿	✿
Obesity			✿	✿
Pregnancy	✿	✿		
Stress	✿	✿	✿	✿

Salabhasana	Setu bandhasana	Chakrasana	Matsyasana	Janu sirsasana	Paschimottanasana	Purvottanasana	Baddha konasana	Upavista konasana	Sukhasana twist	Marichyasana II	Jathara parivartanasana	Sarvangasana	Halasana	Savasana	Viparita karani	Surya namaskar	Ujjayi	Nadi shodhana	Meditation
●			●	●				●								●	●	●	
	●		●	●	●							●				●	●	●	
●	●	●					●					●				●	●	●	
●		●	●				●	●	●	●				●				
●	●	●	●	▲	▲										●	●	●	▲
	●	●	●	●			●	●				●					●	
			●	●		●	●					●	●	●		●		
●	●						●	●									●	●	
	▲	▲	●	●									●					
			●	●			●	●				●	●	●	●		●	
	●		●	●	●		●	●				●	●		●	●	●	
							●		●								●	
	●	●	●	●			●	●		●		●	●		●	●	●	
▲	▲		●	●		●	●				▲	▲	●			●	●	
●	●		●	●		●		●				●	●	●		●	●	●
●	●	●	●									●	●				●	
			●		●	●												
●	●	●	●			●					●	●	●		●	●	●	

Glossary

ADHO MUKHA SVANASANA Downward-facing dog pose

AHIMSA Non-violence, fundamental element of yogic philosophy

ASANA Yoga pose

BADDHA KONASANA Cobbler's pose

BALASANA Child pose

BHUJANGASANA Cobra pose

BHUJAPIDASANA Arm pressure pose

CHAKRA One of seven energy points along the spine, storehouses for prana

CHAKRASANA Wheel pose

CHITTA-VRTTI Fluctuations of the mind

GOMUKHASANA Cow-face pose

HALASANA Plough pose

JANU SIRSASANA Head beyond the knee pose

JATHARA PARIVARTANASANA Stomach-strengthening pose

KARNAPIDASANA Ear pressure pose

KIRLIAN PHOTOGRAPHY Used to record electrical discharge (or 'aura' emitted by humans or objects)

KOSHA Defence against disease

MAKRASANA Crocodile pose

MANTRA Word or phrase repeated as an aid to meditation

MARICHYASANA II Sage twist

MATSYASANA Fish pose

NADI SHODHANA PRANAYAMA Alternate nostril breathing

NADIS Subtle energy meridians

NAVASANA Boat pose

PADMASANA Lotus pose

PARSVAKONASANA Side angle stretch

PARSVOTTANASANA Chest to leg extension

PASCHIMOTTANASANA Stretch on the body's west side

PERFECT POSTURE Standing posture in which the body is balanced

PRANA The body's life force

PRANAYAMA Pranic capacity; control of the prana

PRASARITA PADOTTANASANA Wide leg stretch

PURVOTTANASANA Stretch on the body's east side

REIKI Healing therapy based on the transfer of universal energy

SALABHASANA Locust pose

SAMASTHITI Equal pose

SARVANGASANA Shoulderstand

SAVASANA Corpse pose

SETU BANDHASANA Bridge pose

SHODHANA Purification

SUKHASANA Cross-legged twist

SURYA NAMASKAR Sun salutation

SWASTIKASANA Folded leg pose

TRIANGA MUKHAIKAPADA PASCHIMOTTANASANA Three-limbed forward bend

TRIKONASANA Triangle pose

UJJAYI PRANAYAMA Style of yogic breathing

UPAVISTA KONASANA Seated wide angle pose

UTTANASANA Intense forward stretch

VAJARASANA Firm meditation pose

VEDAS Compilation of early Indian spiritual writings

VIPARITA KARANI Exercise that reverses circulation

VIRABHADRASANA Warrior pose

VISUALISATION Meditation aid in which the postures are recreated in the mind

YOGA-SUTRA Early yoga text

Useful Addresses

YOGA BIOMEDICAL CENTRE AND TRUST

4th Floor, 60 Great Ormond Street,
London WC1N 3HR
Tel: (020 7) 419 7195

YOGA FOR HEALTH FOUNDATION

UK and worldwide HQ
Ickwell Bury
Biggleswade
Bedfordshire,
SG18 9EF
Tel: 01767 627271
Fax: 01767 627266

THE BRIGHTON NATURAL HEALTH CENTRE

27 Regent Street
Brighton BN1 1UL
Tel: (01273) 600 0010

BRITISH WHEEL OF YOGA

1 Hamilton Place
Boston Road
Stamford
Lincolnshire NG34 7ES
Tel: 01529 306851
www.members.aol.com/
wheelyoga

SIVANANDA YOGA VEDANTA CENTRE

51 Felsham Road,
London SW15
Tel: (020 8) 780 0160

DIVINE LIFE SOCIETY

Shivananddear
PT Tehri-Garhwal
Uttar Pradesh
India

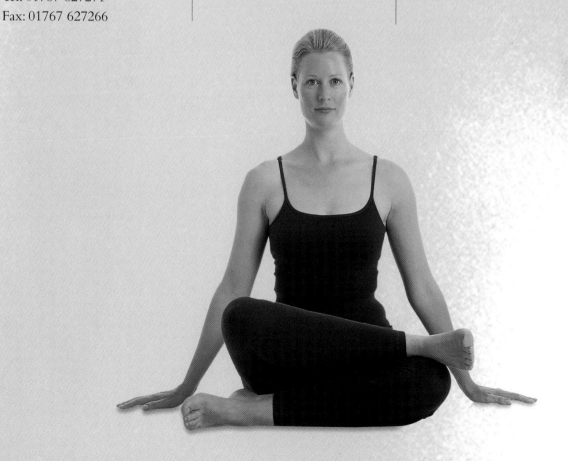

Index

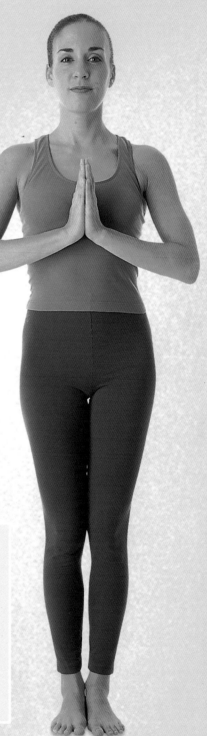

Acknowledgements

Special thanks go to
Franz Andrini, Emma Barton,
Nandhitha Ramaprasad, Jenny
Vanneufville, Christina Brown,
for help with photography

*The publishers would like to thank
the following for the use of pictures:*
Corbis Images 9, 10/11, 15, 59, 88
Image Bank 42/43, 87
Stockmarket 90/91
Stone Gettyone 1, 6/7, 19,
64, 69, 80